D1062507

A PRACTICAL MEDICO-LEGAL GUIDE FOR THE PHYSICIAN

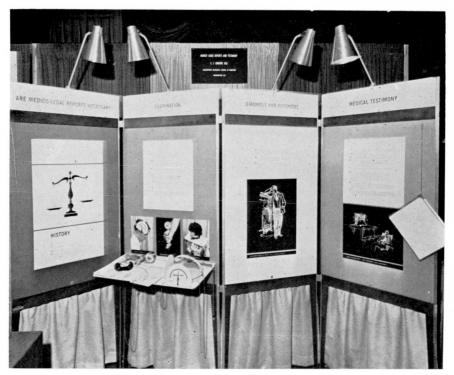

Photograph of Medico-Legal Exhibit.

Scientific exhibit of author, first shown at the American Academy of Orthopaedic Surgeons in Chicago, January 1966. Table contains working models of the Cervigon measurement set and Jamar grip tester, Goniometer, tape measure, tuning fork, Crowe anesthesiometer, and reflex hammer, indicating objective methods of examination. Hanging from chain on right is a sample copy of a typical medico-legal report as suggested.

A PRACTICAL MEDICO-LEGAL GUIDE FOR THE PHYSICIAN

By

EVERETT J. GORDON, M.D., F.A.C.S., F.I.C.S.
Clinical Associate Professor
Georgetown University
School of Medicine
Washington, D.C.

With a Foreword by
THE HONORABLE WILLIAM E. STEWART, JR.
Judge, Superior Court of the District of Columbia

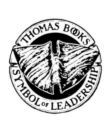

RA
1053
.G65

CHARLES C THOMAS • PUBLISHER
Springfield • Illinois • U.S.A.

INDIANA UNIVERSITY LIBRARY
JUL 11 1979
NORTHWEST

Published and Distributed Throughout the World by
CHARLES C THOMAS • PUBLISHER
BANNERSTONE HOUSE
301-237 East Lawrence Avenue, Springfield, Illinois, U.S.A.

This book is protected by copyright. No
part of it may be reproduced in any manner
without written permission from the publisher.

© *1973, by* CHARLES C THOMAS • PUBLISHER
ISBN 0-398-02688-2

Library of Congress Catalog Card Number: 72-88477

With THOMAS BOOKS *careful attention is given to all details of
manufacturing and design. It is the Publisher's desire to present books
that are satisfactory as to their physical qualities and artistic possibilities
and appropriate for their partcular use.* THOMAS BOOKS *will be true
to those laws of quality that assure a good name and good will.*

Printed in the United States of America

EE-11

hcm
7-11-79

This book is dedicated to the memory of my parents
who made my education possible
and to my brother, Leon S. Gordon, M.D., Ph.D
whose faith and guidance provided the inspiration for my medical
career.

FOREWORD

The author's experience and knowledge in the area of medico-legal examinations and testimony is quite apparent. Much of the distaste, concern and even fright of the uninitiated physician for courtroom appearances can be eliminated by a reading of this book.

This should be a textbook for medical and legal students, both of whom approach the practice of their respective professions completely lacking an appreciation in this area where the professions so often clash.

The value of the author's effort is, however, by no means limited to the beginner in either of the professions. It can be fairly said that many lawyers and physicians, with years of practice to their credit, can indeed profit from the use of this book which combines expertise and practicality.

Exhaustive treatment and reasoned explanations as presented herein will undoubtedly promote a better understanding between the members of the two great professions of medicine and law.

WILLIAM E. STEWART, JR.
Judge
Superior Court of the District of Columbia

vii

PREFACE

This book was written because of the obvious need for more extensive education of physicians in the field of medico-legal medicine. The stimulus for the book arose from the favorable reception given a pamphlet entitled "Medico-Legal Examinations, Reports, and Testimony" which was prepared for a scientific exhibit at the annual convention of the American Academy of Orthopaedic Surgeons in Chicago in January 1966.[12]

Considerable interest was manifested at this convention by the attending orthopaedists and the supply of booklets was quickly exhausted. Requests for copies were received from Canada, Mexico, and all sections of the United States. Many physicians returned to their home communities and showed their copy to their confreres, who promptly wrote for copies for their own use. Fellow members of partnerships and clinic groups desired personal copies. Teaching physicians wrote and asked for sufficient copies to distribute to their resident staff. Industrial clinics and claim departments of large industrial organizations requested copies for their physicians and offered to pay for the material. A personal friend, a prominent congressman who was previously a practicing attorney, forwarded the material to his nephew practicing law in another state. Doctors of all specialties were interested, many of whom had not seen the exhibit but whose attention had been directed to the pamphlet by orthopaedists returning from the convention. Medical societies requested copies for their members and offered to pay for a large number of copies for distribution to them.

Medical magazines evinced a definite interest and requested permission to use quotations in their publications, such as *Medical Economics, Modern Medicine, Health Bulletin* and the *Medical Tribune*. Long distance calls were received from the legal department of General Motors among others for literature and copies of other publications by the author on similar subjects.

Several attorneys wrote asking that a price be quoted for several copies of the pamphlet. In all such instances the pamphlets were sent without charge. Former classmates, from whom the doctor had not heard for years, saw the publication and wrote to express their favorable comments. Several requests were received from the heads of medical school departments which indicated an increased interest in a subject which had long been underemphasized and unexplored. It became apparent that the necessity for improved education in the management and treatment of medico-legal matters, as well as subjects of more clinical interest, was becoming recognized. The article in *Medical Tribune Magazine* mentioned the Cervigon apparatus, which was just being placed on the market; the author has had no association with the distribution of this apparatus although he did aid in its development.

One physician, who was preparing a book on "My Experience on the Witness Stand," commented on the author's experience with medico-legal examinations and was granted permission to use quotes from the pamphlet in his proposed book. An unusual inquiry was received from an international missionary organization which requested numerous copies to be sent to their physicians stationed around the world, demonstrating the need for understanding of medico-legal problems everywhere, not only in the United States where such litigation is more prevalent.

Many orthopaedists expressed interest in this subject, in contrast to some physicians who reject the subject of medico-legal medicine as mundane, and prefer to talk of their recent "total hip prosthesis operation." Undoubtedly these doctors will be involved with many more medico-legal matters than total hip operations or similar operations. Whether they recognize it or not, they must become better versed in the subject if they wish to give their patients the best possible medical service.

A few excerpts from letters received are as follows:

I was fortunate to have the opportunity to read your treatise, "Medico-Legal Examinations, Reports, and Testimony."
I borrowed same from a doctor here at Norristown, who of course, would like it returned to him. If you would be kind enough to forward me

another copy of same so that we may keep it with our permanent records, it would be greatly appreciated.

From a Kentucky orthopaedist:

I just want to tell you that I enjoyed very much your exhibit with regard to "Medico-Legal Examinations, Reports, and Testimony," at the recent Academy meeting in Chicago. You have set forth in your pamphlet very straightforward essentials of examination, reports and testimony. I failed to pick up an extra copy of this for my partner and would appreciate it very much if you would be able to send me a pamphlet for him.

From an Iowa orthopaedist:

Would it be possible to secure another copy of "Medico-Legal Examinations, Reports, and Testimony" written by you?
I would be very happy to reimburse you for same.

From a plaintiff attorney in the District of Columbia:

This article is most excellent and I wish to compliment you on it. It certainly goes a long way in providing the necessary bridge between lawyers and doctors and I would like a couple of extra copies, if you have them, for other lawyers in Virginia.

From a New York radiologist:

I have read with great interest your pamphlet "Medico-Legal Examinations, Reports, and Testimony."
Your excellent covering of the subject has given me valuable information which I will be able to use. As a radiologist, I am quite often called upon to testify in court.
I would greatly appreciate your letting me know where the assignment and authorization forms reprinted in your pamphlet can be obtained.

From a Canadian orthopaedist:

This type of examination and report is of particular interest to me, as I am involved in a great many medico-legal questions. I wonder if you have presented any papers on this topic, or if you have any written material that was used in conjunction with this presentation that I might have for a comparison of methods, and possible improvement of my present format.

Copies of the paper were distributed to several attorneys in the Washington metropolitan area specializing in both plaintiff and defendant representation. Many comments were received, among which were the following from a defendant attorney, later appointed to the federal bench:

I am very impressed with what I have seen and I am sure this is going to be both practical and very worthwhile.

From a prominent plaintiff attorney:
    I have already found it to be a most helpful tool in handling matters in the negotiation and litigation stage.

    This book represents an amplification of the 1966 pamphlet with inclusion of many personal experiences and those of other physicians. The incidents referred to represent actual experiences, but all dates, names, and places have been changed. Any similarity to cases known to the reader is purely coincidental.

                                                                    E.J.G.

CONTENTS

Page

FOREWORD—The Honorable William E. Stewart, Jr. vii

PREFACE ix

1. INTRODUCTION 3

2. MEDICO-LEGAL EXAMINATION AND REPORTS 7

   METHOD OF EXAMINATION 11

   HISTORY 12

   EXAMINATION 26

      A. Physical Examination—General Notes 30

      B. Extremities 37

      C. Grip Testing 38

      D. Cervical Spine 41

      E. Lower Extremities 46

      F. Back—Diagnostic Tests 47

         Functional Manifestations in the Lower Back

         Aids to Differential Diagnosis of Acute Low Back Syndrome

   X-RAYS 64

      Reports of Previous X-Rays 75

      Loss of Lordotic Curve by X-Ray 75

      X-Rays in Children 77

      Hypertrophic Changes—Osteoarthritis 79

      Value of X-Rays in Defendant Examinations 80

      Myelograms 82

   DEFENDANT'S EXAMINATIONS 83

      Obnoxious Patients 84

      Harassment of Defendant Examiner 89

      Scheduling Appointments for Defendant Examinations 96

   DIAGNOSIS 100

      Interpretation of Clinical Findings 101

      Functional Symptoms 104

      Evaluation of Pain 105

      Evaluation of Electroencephalograms 109

      Malingering 110

Orthopaedic Examination of the Malingerer
Full Disclosure of All Diagnoses and Objective Findings
3. TREATMENT 120
   MEDICATION AND DUPLICATE PRESCRIPTIONS 120
   PHYSICAL THERAPY 121
   HOME CARE 125
   PHYSICAL THERAPY AS AN AID IN DIAGNOSIS 126
   OFFICE TREATMENT AND EXERCISE FORMS 127
   HOSPITALIZATION 136
   SURGERY—SIGNIFICANCE IN MEDICO-LEGAL
      CASES 144
   REPORTS CONCERNING SURGICAL PROCEDURES 152
   PROGNOSIS 164
4. MEDICAL REPORTS 171
   FORMAT 171
      A. Plaintiff Reports 173
      B. Defendant Reports 176
   PROGRESS REPORTS 184
   AVAILABILITY OF HOSPITAL RECORDS 190
   REVIEW OF MEDICAL REPORTS FOR DEFENDANT
      EXAMINATION 191
   ALTERATION OF REPORTS 192
   FORWARDING OF REPORTS 193
5. FEES 197
   FEE SCHEDULES 197
   ASSIGNMENTS 199
      A. For Attorney 199
      B. For Medical Pay Coverage 202
   PERIODIC STATUS REPORTS 204
   HEALTH AND ACCIDENT INSURANCE—
      ASSIGNMENTS 207
   MEDICAL PAY COVERAGE 212
   FALSE INFORMATION REGARDING ATTORNEY
      REPRESENTATION 215
   BILLING PROCEDURE 216
   DETERMINATION OF FEES FOR TESTIMONY 217
   FEES FOR DEFENDANT TESTIMONY AND
      EXAMINATIONS 223
   FEES FOR DEPOSITIONS 225
   PRE-PAYMENT OF FEES FOR TESTIMONY 226

TESTIMONY IN RESPONSE TO SUBPOENA
WITHOUT FEE AGREEMENT 226
ACCEPTANCE OF REDUCED FEES 227

6. QUALIFICATIONS 230

7. TESTIMONY 232
IMPORTANCE AND VALUE 232
MANNER AND TIME OF TESTIMONY 234
SUBPOENA AS ORDINARY WITNESS 239
SIGNIFICANCE OF VOLUNTARY AGREEMENT
TO TESTIFY 246
CONTEMPT OF COURT FOR FAILURE TO COM-
PLY WITH SUBPOENA 247
PRE-TRIAL CONFERENCE WITH ATTORNEY 248
TESTIMONY REGARDING MALINGERING 248
INTRODUCTION OF SURPRISE MEDICAL EVIDENCE .249
USE OF EXHIBITS 250
MEDICAL RECORDS IN THE COURTROOM 252
X-RAYS—BRING THEM TO COURT! 252
REVIEW OF PRIOR X-RAYS 254
TESTIMONY—CONFLICT WITH MEDICAL CON-
VENTIONS AND VACATIONS 255
RELATIVE WEIGHT OF TESTIMONY OF
SPECIALISTS 258
TESTIMONY—FULL DISCLOSURE OF ALL EV-
IDENCE 260
TESTIMONY ON BEHALF OF OPPOSING COUNSEL 263
INTERVENTION OF JUDGES 265
IMPARTIAL MEDICAL TESTIMONY 267
DEPOSITION 269
DEPOSITION USED FOR HARASSMENT 275

8. CROSS-EXAMINATION 279
BASIS AND TECHNIQUES 279
RECOGNITION OF TEXT BOOKS AS AUTHORITIES ... 283
INCONSISTENCY OF TESTIMONY WITH PREVI-
OUS TESTIMONY OR MEDICAL PUBLICATIONS
OF WITNESS 285
OBSERVATION OF OPPOSING ATTORNEY 293
MISQUOTES 294
ALLEGED INCONSISTENCIES IN MEDICAL
REPORTS 295

HARASSMENT BY A "FRIENDLY ATTORNEY" 298
INSERTION OF EVIDENCE 301
REACTION TO ABUSE 303
HELPFUL POINTERS FOR CROSS-EXAMINATION 305
9. USEFUL LEGAL FORMS AND PRINTED INSTRUC-
TIONS 315
10. CONCLUSION 318
BIBLIOGRAPHY 326
ILLUSTRATIONS 329
INDEX 331

A PRACTICAL MEDICO-LEGAL GUIDE FOR THE PHYSICIAN

1 INTRODUCTION

To the average physician, medico-legal proceedings are a hazy aspect of practice that he would like to forget and ignore, and that he hopes will "pass him by." He fails to recognize that the complexity of modern living not only affects our health, but increasingly involves numerous problems and disputes which require a legal or judicial process for settlement or resolution. The practicing physician must have some familiarity with legal problems, in addition to his formal medical training, in order to present testimony in a legal proceeding or to write a proper report, both of which may materially affect the final decision. He must be trained to understand and evaluate the interest of the individuals involved in these sometimes complex problems.

The need for medico-legal education has been repeatedly stressed by both physicians and attorneys. At present there are no major programs in the United States for training physicians in medico-legal trial work, even though 68 per cent of all trial level cases in the United States courts involve medical evidence. These figures were recently given by William J. Currans, Professor of Health Law at Harvard Medical School, who also made several suggestions for teaching legal and social values to medical students. The increasing importance of a medical witness has been recognized by the periodic medico-legal symposia sponsored by the American Bar Association and American Medical Association, the introduction of instructional courses in medico-legal procedure at the annual convention of the American Academy of Orthopaedic Surgeons, and the formation of the American College of Legal Medicine.

3

A physician in active practice will probably be involved in a legal proceeding at some time in his medical career; he should prepare himself to make his participation both competent and helpful. This book is an effort to improve his role as an expert witness and to aid him in formulating and expressing a medical opinion in a properly prepared report. The reluctance of physicians to become professional witnesses is often attributable to their lack of information or instruction and proper guidance. It is hoped that this book will enable physicians to fulfill this obligation to their patients impartially and without apprehension. In many communities only a small group of physicians regularly participate in medico-legal matters; unfortunately some of these physicians do not properly represent the medical profession because of their bias and obvious advocacy for either the plaintiff or the defendant. With increased participation by competent physicians the medical image should be improved and enhanced; this will be reflected in a more cooperative and favorable attitude by judges, lawyers, and the various communications media.

Contact with some aspect of a legal process is an inescapable part of a physician's professional life, emanating from the patient-physician relationship. Irrespective of the personal desires of either party, a controverted legal action involving medical issues can only be resolved by expert medical opinion, offered in either written or oral form by attending or consulting physicians. Frequently the physician is the most important witness at a trial, especially if the question of liability is clear or uncontested. The physician must state the correct diagnosis of the injured patient and also outline a complete prognosis in regard to permanence of physical impairment, diminished earning capacity, continued pain and suffering, need of further medical attention, life expectancy, cosmetic disfigurement, and other factors. People of all income levels have access to legal aid, either through private attorneys or charitable agencies and legal aid programs from the local bar associations. The contingency arrangement prevailing throughout the United States is often cited as a great advantage to the poor, permitting them to avail themselves of competent legal talent which would otherwise be denied to those unable to afford such services.

There has been a definite trend in our social legislation to expand the legislative social benefits to greater segments of our population, resulting in legal processes requiring medical assistance for resolution. A medical opinion is frequently required when a patient or his representative attempts to secure financial benefits from a federal, state, municipal or private agency or from private individuals.

In Europe the adversary system is not widely established, and a greater reliance is placed upon depositions, without extensive court appearances. In contrast, the American system of law frequently requires the active participation of the physician in a trial proceeding.

Categories of legal action requiring medical opinion from physicians in this country, include the following:

1. Workmen's Compensation insurance cases, which may involve litigation against private insurance carriers, the federal government, Longshoremen's Act, etc.
2. Personal injury suits instituted under common and statutory law.
3. Insurance contract disputes for determination of permanent disability or total disability in health and accident policies, the establishment of the necessity for continued medical care within policy limits such as in medical payment policies on automobiles, or determination of cause of death in life insurance policies.
4. Qualification for social security disability and benefits, death benefits for employees of federal, state, and municipal agencies.
5. Retirement of Civil Service employees for disability. This constitutes a large segment of contested medical opinion for retirement for medical disability, as it awards the employee a tax-free benefit but does not prevent him from working elsewhere in a different or similar occupation.
6. Qualification for licensure for automobile, driving permits, airplane pilot permits.
7. Qualification for a rehabilitation program such as the vocational rehabilitation programs of federal and state agencies.
8. Miscellaneous medical problems such as resolution of contested wills, confirmation of income tax deductions for medical expenses, testimony in criminal action resulting in personal injury or death, excuses from work for medical reasons, medical evidences in divorce proceedings, alimony payments, etc.

9. Medical reports pertaining to military service. Medical opinions are frequently requested with regard to both entry and discharge from military service, or to establish medical disabilities for such service. The physician is frequently asked to examine a prospective draftee and report his medical findings for exclusion from the draft or for limited military service because of medical disability. Those in military service must be properly evaluated by a military physician prior to discharge to establish percentages of medical disability and eligibility for retirement.

To such problems that involve legal action dependent on clinical findings and medical opinion, we now turn our attention.

2 MEDICO-LEGAL EXAMINATIONS AND REPORTS

A GOOD MEDICAL REPORT IN A CASE INVOLVING LITIGATION IS VITAL TO A FAIR SETTLEMENT AND RECOVERY OF DAMAGES BY THE CLAIMANT. BOTH THE PLAINTIFF AND DEFENDANT ATTORNEYS MUST HAVE A COMPLETE AND UNBIASED DESCRIPTION AND PROGNOSIS OF THE INJURIES SUSTAINED BY THE PATIENT IN ORDER TO EVALUATE THEIR CASES PROPERLY AND DECIDE UPON A MONETARY AWARD. ONLY THE PHYSICIAN WHO HAS EXAMINED THE PATIENT CAN PROVIDE THE NECESSARY MEDICAL INFORMATION.[12,19]

If the physician does not wish to become involved in a medico-legal matter, he should notify the patient immediately, at the initial visit, that he does not wish to assume responsibility for his care and prefers to withdraw from the case. Once he has made an examination, he is subject to subpoena and is then legally bound to submit a medical report, if necessary by legal deposition or court testimony. The physician who is unwilling to prepare a proper report or testify on behalf of his patient should promptly inform him of that fact if the clinical history has disclosed the possible medico-legal nature of the case. At this point the physician should decide whether or not he wishes to undertake treatment of this patient, realizing that he is legally obligated not only to provide proper medical care but also to prepare reports and give medical testimony should he continue with the case.

Medico-legal examinations involve more detail than the usual examination of a patient who presents himself solely for diagnosis and treatment. Not only must a physician concern himself with all facets of the history, but he must methodically record the information in every detail. For this purpose the use of dictating apparatus is essential; the examiner may record the history and the various physical findings in the presence of the patient, but it may be wise to defer dictating his professional opinion and prognosis until the patient has departed. Prefabricated forms may be used to record his objective findings, such as outlines of examinations of the neck and low back, or a chart showing comparative ranges of motion in the examination of the hand and fingers.

In a defendant examination the doctor should make notes as he proceeds, using charts to record various tests and comparative measurements, instead of dictating what might be negative findings in the hearing of the patient. The physician will thus avoid arousing resentment in a hostile plaintiff who may have submitted to a defendant examination against his will.

Some physicians disdainfully reject medico-legal examinations whenever possible in preference to more glamorous surgery and hospital care. When it becomes necessary for them to perform such examinations, they do so superficially and as rapidly as possible, and often write an all too brief report. Although they may be excellent surgeons and astute physicians, their apparent competence will more than likely be rated by their examination of and report on a patient involved in some personal injury litigation. The author has often heard patients express derogatory remarks about well-known, competent surgeons of high professional rank because of the cursory nature of their medico-legal examination. These patients may not return to such a surgeon for a surgical procedure, despite his demonstrated professional skill, because of their misinterpretation of his competency as reflected in his examination.

The type of patient who states his symptoms fairly and honestly, with no attempt to exaggerate, may remark to the defendant examiner that his own physician had never taken as thorough a medical history or performed as detailed a physical examination, including comparative measurements, as that being carried out by the consultant for the defense. The patient may report that his doctor had only partially undressed him, "poked him a bit," and spent only a few minutes in the examination.

Patients are prone to exaggerate in this respect and perhaps will make the same criticism of you if there appears to be some basis for their remarks. On the other hand, the patient may complain to the defendant consultant that he would undoubtedly be feeling better and would not have his persistent subjective complaints had he come to him initially for treatment.

In one such incident, a registered nurse asked the defendant physician whether he practiced in her suburban area, stating that there were no competent orthopaedists in that suburb. After she had been informed that there were in fact several reputable orthopaedists practicing in that vicinitiy, she stated that she had consulted two of them and neither one had made as thorough an examination as he did. This example demonstrates how a patient judges professional competency, on the detail of the doctor's examination rather than other professional skills. Such situations arise because otherwise competent physicians have little interest in medico-legal matters and perform limited examinations, under the mistaken preconceived impression that the individual who comes for consultation is really not very sick and a full examination is not required for diagnosis or treatment.

Physicians who have a large practice, and who have established a reputation for competency in medico-legal matters, occasionally encounter a former patient who has had a second or third injury, either as a plaintiff or a defendant. In either case, it is helpful if the patient is identified as having previously visited that office; the patient's past record can be consulted and helpful information obtained. However, the patient may have forgotten his previous visit and both the receptionist and the doctor may fail to recognize him. The doctor may have moved to a new office in a different locality, and the patient may forget he had visited the same doctor at his former location. He will have additional difficulty in recognition if the doctor has changed his appearance, such as "adopting the new look" with a beard, long hair, moustache, long sideburns, and so on. The alert, observant physician ought to remember the patient by sight or by name; he can then consult his previous records as this may be of value in his treatment as well as in evaluating the medical examination.

A patient whose chart indicated definite anxiety and continued complaints despite all forms of treatment would require a different plan of treatment from that of the stoical type, who is anxious to have his treatment completed so that he can return to work as early as possible. The records may also reflect effective medical agents in treating that patient, which would shorten the period of medical care. For example, a patient who previously had injuries to his neck and back, but also exhibited a considerable anxiety overlay, had received several tranquilizing agents over an extensive time interval. He had been treated approximately eight years previously after a similar accident, and had received an abundance of physical therapy without response. Tranquilizing medication had been only partially effective, and it was only with great difficulty that the patient finally returned to his job as a printer. Eventually his symptoms cleared after cessation of treatment and the firm reassurance that he had no residual disability. When the patient returned after the second accident, he again continued to complain despite objective improvement in his condition. This time, in spite of his complaints, tranquilizers were not prescribed and he was returned to work at an early date; his subjective complaints completely cleared without need of further treatment.

Recall of a previous visit is especially important in the examination for a defendant. Occasionally, the plaintiff will not mention in his medical history any facts relating to his previous examination, either having forgotten his visit to that doctor, or having remembered and hoping that the doctor will not recognize him. If he denies any previous injuries or accidents, this can be incorporated into the report and will represent important evidence relating to the patient's veracity, with a corresponding impression on the court. In one instance, a clear-cut case of liability loss resulted in a defendant's verdict because of just this type of demonstrated evidence of a patient's prevarication. More importantly, the examining doctor is in a better position to size up the patient's complaints if he has previously evaluated him and has a record of the objective evidence as related to that individual's subjective complaints. In addition, x-rays from a previous examination of the same areas, such as a second injury to his neck, may be available, which would be valuable to the examiner for evaluation of pre-existing degenerative changes, arthritis, reversal of normal curvatures, etc.

METHOD OF EXAMINATION

A medico-legal examination consists of a complete history, a careful, detailed physical examination, and x-rays as indicated. The history should be regarded as an important part of the examination; sometimes a patient who is being examined on behalf of the defendant is under the misconception that there will be only a physical examination and that he need not tell the doctor what part of the body was injured or give any medical history whatsoever. Obviously, it is difficult to evaluate the injuries sustained without knowledge of what area was injured, how the accident occurred (mechanism of injury), what treatment was administered and its results, present complaints and present disability, as well as past medical history. This situation usually occurs when the patient has been erroneously advised by his attorney to give no information whatsoever to the defendant's examining physician, suggesting the "name, rank and serial number" instructions of a prisoner of war!

Examinations performed on behalf of either the plaintiff or defendant should be essentially similar, but the final discussion in a defendant medical report should avoid recommendations for treatment. The medical history in a defendant examination should be more detailed regarding previous injuries, accidents and medical problems, current treatment, frequency of medical visits, and disability for work. Sometimes the examining physician has been alerted by the defendant to make a detailed inquiry regarding previous injuries or accidents. This procedure may help to determine the veracity of the patient, especially if he denies previous accidents of which the defendant is aware through a central index registry. If the patient denies facts which are already known to the examining physician through review of verified records, his veracity and credibility are certainly open to question and should be considered when evaluating his continuing subjective symptoms and complaints. Usually such "lapses of memory" occur without the knowledge or approval of the patient's attorney, who is well aware of the adverse impact of a suddenly exposed false history on a jury. A defendant's verdict is not uncommon in such cases, even with clear liability.

HISTORY

The medical history is an integral part of all medical examinations. An accurate, detailed history will often indicate a presumptive diagnosis to an experienced examiner even before he performs the physical portion of the examination. A history is necessary before any treatment other than emergency care can be administered, as well as in an evaluation of the subjective complaints and present physical condition of the patient, whether due to illness or injury. The history may be either brief or lengthy and involved, depending upon the time interval from the date of onset of complaints or injury until the examination is performed. If there has been a clear-cut physical injury such as a fracture without complications, the history is usually concise and easily taken; however, if the complaints are based on a strong emotional or nervous overlay which has resulted in numerous consultations, switching of physicians, considerable treatment—physical therapy, surgical or medical, the history is apt to be very extensive and require more than the usual time to obtain. The nervous type of patient often wishes to talk and ramble in relating his or her problems to the doctor and may have to be interrupted in order to clarify particular details. This type of patient also tends to repeat herself and reiterate various versions of the same complaints.

A complete history should be taken on every personal injury case. It should begin with current complaints, but should also include any initial injuries which have healed in the interim between the accident and the examination. Defense examinations are often delayed until several months, or even years, after the injuries were sustained, and some of the initial complaints will have subsided. The report should include information regarding the manner of injury, such as a fall down steps or on a sidewalk, a pedestrian accident, an auto accident, an altercation, or a boat accident, etc. The date and time of accident, street or road location, or general locality should be stated. If the accident involved an auto collision, the statement should identify the size and type of vehicles involved, such as standard-sized vehicle, small foreign car, truck, bus, tractor trailer, etc. This is definitely important as one would anticipate more injuries to the occupants of a Volkswagen struck by a large Greyhound bus than to passengers in the bus struck by a Volkswagen! Trucks vary considerably in size, from small panel trucks the size of a large passenger sedan, to gasoline trailers, concrete mixers, large interstate van trucks, etc. Obviously the impact from a massive loaded tractor trailer could be assumed to be greater than that from a small delivery panel truck.

Further details should be obtained as to where the patient was sitting in the automobile, whether he was wearing a seat belt or shoulder harness, and what his position was relative to the point of impact; these details should also reflect the type of collision, whether rear-end with the car stopped or a moving collision, giving some idea of the relative force of the impact. In a major collision with serious injuries, the patient should be asked whether or not he was thrown out of the car onto the pavement, or whether he struck the dashboard, windshield, steering wheel, sun visor, or side of the car. Further information as to whether the patient was thrown from one side of the car to the other, or thrown from the rear seat on to the floor or against the rear or the front seat, should also be obtained. This type of information is more important in the report than trying to ascertain whose fault it was the accident occurred, who went through the red light, and other details which should not be included in the doctor's medical history.

Inquiries should be made as to where the patient went directly after the accident. If he continued to work and did not consult a doctor until the next day or several days later, the type of injury could be assumed to be less severe than if he was removed by ambulance, police car, or another driver, directly to a hospital emergency room. This is not absolutely true as the officials on the scene may wish to have the individuals involved in the accident examined at a hospital as a precautionary measure. It is important to know whether the injured person was able to get out of the car without help or whether he was taken out by stretcher. Other important information concerns loss of consciousness, loss of memory for details of the accident, and occurrence of blackout spells.

A brief past medical history should always be taken with particular reference to accidental injuries and previous auto or motorcycle accidents. Surgical procedures should be reported with dates and hospital where performed, in order to provide a record for further inquiry if necessary. A brief summary of previous medical problems is important; this should include nervous problems, cardiac disease, spastic colitis, "nervous stomach," and other ailments, any of which may give a clue to the general make-up of the individual being examined.

The patient should also be asked about previous accidents with personal injury litigation. If he has had a similar type of injury in the past, it should be determined whether or not this case had been closed and a good recovery made from that accident, with no recurrence of symptoms dating prior to the present accident. Although some plaintiff attorneys will object to inclusion of this information, it is pertinent to a complete evaluation of the injuries sustained; the defendant's insurance company will probably discover these facts anyway, especially if the case warrants a thorough investigation. Such a listing of facts regarding prior litigation will identify the examiner as being impartial and fair in his appraisal of the injured party.

Many details of the history can be taken by the receptionist and noted on the chart (Figure 1). The doctor should then review these with the patient and amplify the record as indicated. If the patient states that the history was taken solely by the receptionist, it is important that the doctor have a personal knowledge of the details; otherwise it will be considered *hearsay evidence* and will not be admissible in testimony. Once the facts are recorded by his receptionist, it will only take a few moments for the doctor to review them briefly with the patient. The history will be much

NAME:
ADDRESS:

TEL:
PRESENT EMPLOYER:
OCCUPATION:
ADDRESS:

TEL: EXT:

INITIAL VISIT: DATE _____
Place: Off. Hosp. _____

COMPLAINT OR INITIAL INJURY:

DURATION:

HISTORY OF PRESENT ILLNESS:

D/A: / / , a.m.   p.m.
PLACE: _____
X-RAYS: _____
    Date:
    Place:
HOSPITAL VISITED _____
STOPPED WORK: _____

TREATMENT:

Age: _____ Sex ____ Birthplace _____ Birthdate _____

MARITAL STATUS _____ Div. Date _____

NEAREST RELATIVE _____
Relationship _____
Address _____
Tel _____ Occupation _____
Employer _____
Address _____
Tel _____

Medicare or Med Serv _____ Code ____ Subs ____
Other insurance _____
ATTORNEY _____
MED PAY _____ POL.# _____
COMP CARRIER _____
REFERRED BY _____
VS: _____

Driver _____ Passenger _____ Front ____ Rear ____
                                  Right ____ Left ____
Rear End Collison _____ Moving Collision _____

SEAT BELT: YES ____ NO ____
TYPE OF CAR: Pt: _____
        other car _____
BRIEF DETAILS:

DOCTORS SEEN: _____
RETURNED TO WORK _____

PAST MEDICAL HISTORY:

Dislocations, fractures, or injuries

Previous surgery:

Serious medical illnesses, nervous problems, hypertension, allergies, medication

Previous lawsuits or claims for personal injuries
    Settled?

FIGURE 1. HISTORY SHEET.

shorter in the examination of a plaintiff immediately after an accident than in a defendant examination conducted several weeks, months, or even years later. However, the same general format should be followed in all cases.

It may be helpful if the examining physician has some idea of the type of property damage incurred by the patient's vehicle, although there is no inflexible relationship. Occasionally the patient will bring a picture of his damaged vehicle, which then gives the physician a clear idea of how the patient sustained his injuries; the development of any anxiety overlay may be more comprehensible to the physician after seeing such a picture, especially if there are minimal physical injuries. Of course, there are incidences of severe property damage wherein the driver and passengers walk away unharmed, but these are not too common.

The initial treating physician usually has no difficulty in obtaining a full, detailed history, but when the examination is performed on behalf of the defendant, the information may have to be supplied by the defendant or his legal representative if the plaintiff is uncooperative and refuses to answer pertinent questions. Most claimants will give the necessary medical information if the examination is conducted in the proper manner, but inquiries into the details of the accident are often resisted by the patient on instructions from his attorney. If this occurs, difficulty in obtaining additional facts regarding the medical history may result and then further retard the examination.

The defendant doctor may be cross-examined in court upon some elements of the history, such as the type of impact, amount of damages sustained, speed of vehicles involved, etc., especially if he has testified that he found minimal residuals or none as a result of the accident. Should the doctor respond that it would be helpful if he had known such facts as the speed of the cars, exact mode of collision, whether the patient's car was struck on the driver's side, and so on, but is not aware of them, then the opposing attorney may use this "lack of familiarity with the facts" to devaluate and de-emphasize his testimony. The physician may counter this tactic by stating that he is able to testify as to the actual physical condition of the patient at the time of his examination no matter how or when his injuries were sustained. It is generally agreed that the doctor performing a defendant examination should make a limited inquiry into the details and not probe into the legal aspects of the accident in order to establish liability. These factors are considered beyond his domain of interest and may prejudice the value of his medical testimony.

The examiner who has spent the major part of the examination on an analysis of the accident and the patient's background and medical history should not then perform only a minimal physical examination. Such has been the practice of a few physicians specializing almost entirely in medico-legal medicine; plaintiff attorneys often object to that approach in an examiner, and even when it is accepted, the attorneys in the case will carefully instruct their patients not to answer all of the medical examiner's questions. The type of examination here referred to may provide some helpful facts for the accident investigation, but it has limited value for medical evidence. A physician should report the medical history in an impartial manner, without any attempt to establish liability; this last is the obligation of the defendant, not of the doctor making a medical evaluation on his behalf.

Further questions should determine whether or not the patient was unconscious, how he got out of the automobile (under his own power or whether he had to be removed by stretcher), and whether he was able to stand on his feet immediately afterwards. This is important because frequently the accident victim is removed by ambulance or rescue squad directly to a hospital for examination, as directed by standard operating procedures. However, it may be learned that the victim was able to get out of the car and walk over to the ambulance for transfer to the hospital, something which could just as well have been accomplished by police car or private automobile. Thus, transfer of a patient to a nearby hospital by ambulance does not necessarily mean that he was severely injured; the great majority of such cases are not admitted to the hospital after examination in the emergency ward. A few may be retained for several hours for observation, but most accident victims are given first aid, have medication prescribed, and then are released to the care of their private physician. Many of these individuals are only momentarily stunned or "shook up" by the accident and are not actually unconscious, an important clue in the later diagnosis of cerebral concussion.

If the patient is released after a short period of observation in the hospital emergency room, it is probable that he was not seriously injured and did not suffer a definite episode of unconsciousness, as otherwise a competent physician would have detained him for further study; however, in busy emergency centers or understaffed institutions, occasional errors in diagnosis do occur. A correct diagnosis cannot always be made upon immediate examination, but some patients will not remain for prolonged observation because of economic expense, necessity to return to work, or belief they are not hurt. Understandably, some individuals do not wish to wait several hours in an overcrowded emergency room, and leave without being examined.

The doctor should inquire regarding the initial complaints immediately after the accident, as the patient could develop other complaints at a later date, which may be either related or unrelated to the accident, depending on the time of onset. If there is a record of the emergency room visit, it is helpful to note the complaints and diagnoses made at that time as compared to the current complaints. Further information may be obtained by learning of x-rays taken immediately after the accident, and by noting what parts of the body were x-rayed. Usually these correspond to the area of complaint.

Sometimes subsequent inquiry reveals that the patient's complaints are now in an entirely different area of the body than the one x-rayed, indicating either that there were no initial symptoms in that first area or else that the other area of complaint was overlooked. If the later complaints developed several weeks or months after the accident, there may be serious doubt as to the association of that particular complaint with the accident in question. Although it is possible for injuries of the neck and back to demonstrate no significant symptoms until several days or even one or two weeks after the accident, any symptoms which develop after two weeks would be of dubious association. The history should therefore note all of the initial injuries and then the residual complaints which are still causing difficulty.

The examiner should also ascertain whether the patient suffered from anxiety or nervousness immediately after the accident, as this reaction could be responsible for a considerable amount of discomfort and many subjective complaints. Such symptoms may be related to the accident and can be as disabling as serious physical injury, especially if there is a history of pre-existing nervous tension or anxiety, which could have been aggravated by the accident. Prior nervous problems may be indicated by "nervous breakdowns," discharge from military service or refusal of induction on grounds of "nervousness," award of a disability pension by Veterans Administration for mental illness, previous care by psychiatrists or a mental hospital, or persistent medical problems related to peptic ulcers, spastic colon, ulcerative colitis, hypertension, and other symptoms, all of which are known to have a nervous component. Other indications of a nervous problem are mental lapses for recent dates and names when the patient relates his history, or unexplained periods of prolonged idleness, which may be related to mental care. For example, a patient was unemployed for six months prior to the accident and unemployed for a year thereafter. Questioning revealed that he had left his job without apparent reason following nine years of steady employment in his position. Obviously, there was some mental or physical reason for leaving the job prior to the accident which was not related to the accidental injury; this factor also undoubtedly influenced the alleged disability from the accident being litigated.

When fractures or other serious injuries have occurred, the details regarding treatment, administration of antitoxins in compound wounds, antibiotics, length of hospitalization, length of immobilization in casts, splints, follow-up physical therapy, after removal of plaster, patient's response to therapy, period of crutch-walking, etc., should be obtained and noted. Occasionally the patient will bring with him a record of his previous hospitalization, or the doctor may be furnished this information by the patient's attorney. A written record is usually more accurate, as the patient often forgets the details of his medical care, and after a passage of time becomes confused as to dates, length of time cast worn, and so forth. All such details help to determine the period of disability which actually resulted from the injuries sustained. The loss of time from work is important and should include not only the time lost immediately after the accident, but also additional absences at later dates, including visits to the doctor's office and time out for other medical care.

The occupation and type of work performed must be known in order to evaluate the disability resulting from a specific accident. For example, an individual who has a walking cast may be able to perform desk duties but cannot undertake heavy labor, carpenter work, steel erection, and such tasks. The patient's reply regarding time lost from work should be broken down into total or partial disability if possible, but frequently the patient will state he does not remember details as several months have elapsed. Other patients will not give this information on instructions from their attorney.

The physician who is treating an injured person should make notes so that he can report the length of time the patient was off work; these will also provide information for possible court testimony and cross–examination; both total and partial disability should be recorded. After completion of health and accident forms which request the dates of disability, the physician should see that this information is recorded in the patient's chart, preferably with a photocopy of the form. Sometimes the attorney for the defendant will have access to such reports and may use this information to cross-examine the physician. If the latter is not prepared to give an answer similar to that already recorded on the health and accident form, the value of his court testimony will be lowered.

Questions should be asked regarding treatment after the patient's initial visit to the hospital or his physician, and the follow-up care should be briefly summarized. It should be noted especially whether the patient had medical care immediately after the accident or deferred treatment until several weeks or months later, thereby giving a clue to the degree of severity of the initial injury. However, it is recognized that some patients put off going to a physician in the hope that their condition will improve without the necessity of medical care. Thus, although the lack of immediate attention does not necessarily imply that the patient has received no injury, it does usually suggest a relatively minor injury.

The frequency of visits to the physician is significant in this regard: the number of visits should usually diminish gradually as the patient's condition improves. Daily visits for treatment, or "daily except Sunday," are seldom indicated and usually can be stopped after the first five to ten days; whereupon treatment three times a week, then twice a week, then less frequently, is undertaken. The type of treatment received is also important, as frequently patients will state that they received only "heat" treatments without massage, exercises, traction, or other modalities of physical therapy; whereas much of this treatment could easily have been undertaken at home. Prolonged daily visits to a physician (often without treatment on Saturdays and Sundays) make one wonder why not on those days also, if the patient is so sick? Such inconsistency would indicate a possible non-organic basis for the complaints, or even a possible "build-up" of the case by the attending physician. This type of excessive medical care is sometimes encountered in litigation cases, especially when the physician believes his fee is assured regardless of his patient's resources. Such abuses are infrequent, however.

Overtreatment of a medico-legal case may actually cause harm, as unnecessary treatment may bring about a feeling of disability and promote an anxiety neurosis in the patient. By contrast, prompt and correct treatment given only as long as actually needed will restore confidence and stimulate the patient to increased activity and an early return to work; this is beneficial to both the patient's mental and physical health. Not infrequently, patients who have been overtreated remain neurotic cripples even after the litigation has been settled and suffer lifetime disability, never to be compensated by the monetary recovery resulting from their litigation.

The patient should also be questioned with regard to response to treatment—whether treatment helped and the symptoms gradually receded, or the patient's condition persisted. If the symptoms remained unchanged despite continued treatment for many weeks, it would indicate the necessity for a specialist consultation or further examinations to seek another cause or different treatment for the patient's complaints; there would be no value in the continuation of similar therapy, which has been without real benefit to him. A clue to the diagnosis may be given by a detailed review of past medical history, noting the patient's attitude toward his injury and the prospect of returning to work; if he is depressed, pessimistic, reiterating a feeling of disability, he may be subject to anxiety or in a neurotic state, or he may possibly be malingering.

If the patient has been using orthopaedic supports such as a cervical collar, low back corset, or brace, this situation should be evaluated by proper questions. Should the patient state that these supports did not help his condition, yet he continued to use them for several weeks or months, the examiner should be suspicious whether he actually used them or not, and, if he did, inquire why under the circumstances the patient continued to do so. With a true muscle strain, in either the cervical or lumbar areas, some benefit is usually derived from a good support. Frequently, a patient who is not wearing the required brace at the time of the examination, will state that he uses the support every day; the excuse is usually given that he left it at home this particular time to "have it washed." Although this may be true, usually it is not the full explanation, and indicates that the patient is not using the support regularly. The patient may state that he always wears a collar or low back support when riding in an automobile, but that day drove to the doctor's office without it because "I knew I would have to take it off when I got here for the examination." Inasmuch as removing a support represents only a few moments of time and is relatively easy for an individual accustomed to putting it on and taking it off daily, this is not an acceptable answer. In other instances, the patient may wear the garment into the office stating he uses it regularly, and yet inspection shows it to be in practically new condition, with no evidence of having been washed. In addition, the collar or brace may be worn very loosely, giving little or no support.

Sometimes the lack of significant function of the collar can be noted by observing the patient in the waiting room prior to examination, or as he walks into the examining room, perhaps wearing it very loosely with no obvious support resulting from its use. The treating physician who prescribes a support should check its fit before committing the patient to prolonged use, then remove the brace promptly when it is no longer needed in order to avoid dependence upon the support. Prolonged use can cause a mental fixation which hinders removal and discontinuance of the apparatus. A similar situation can arise with a cane or crutches used longer than required.

The history should include a statement from the patient regarding his present condition, such as whether he feels improved, when he feels he will return to work, and so on. This may give some clue as to his mental attitude toward the accident. One patient may state he will be disabled for the rest of his life when obviously this is not true, whereas other patients will state they feel fine, admit improvement, and be ready to resume normal activities. The patient's pessimistic opinion of his ability to return to normal occupational status is often a sign of a functional basis for his continued subjective complaints. If the patient is not working, try to learn the reason for this inactivity, whether it is related to the accident, the result of continuing symptoms, or can be explained by other extraneous factors (unrelated to the accident), such as lack of a job, alcholism, mental problems, social factors or home factors.

The date of the patient's last medical examination or visit should be recorded. In a defendant examination, this visit may have just preceded your examination or may be scheduled the next day, upon advisement of the plaintiff attorney in order to have an evaluation by both the plaintiff and defendant in approximately the same time interval. If this is the case, the approximate dates of preceding visits should be established, as the patient may not have seen his treating physician for several months or a year prior to his recent visit, which was for evaluation only. This time lapse would indicate questionable need of further medical care, and also give information regarding validity of present complaints; obviously, the symptoms of a patient who is complaining as vociferously now as he did two years ago, yet has had no medical care in the interim, must be evaluated with skepticism. If the patient is still under medical care, the examiner should inquire regarding any contemplated surgery, such as plastic surgery, bone grafting, or other surgical procedures, and about plans for hospitalization for diagnosis or therapy, as all of these factors provide additional material for a total evaluation of the case.

In evaluating injuries under Workmen's Compensation law, questions regarding the duration of employment with the present employer may be helpful. Sometimes questioning will elicit information that the employee was just discharged or was unable to get along with his supervisors, or had other personnel clashes, and that this caused the employee to attempt retribution through a medical claim. The individual who remains off work for several weeks or months following a minor accident for which competent treatment was given, after only a few days' employment with that particular firm, should be examined carefully and his complaints carefully evaluated against that background. The examination of such an employee often reflects little or no objective findings to explain his continued subjective symptoms and apparent failure to respond to good treatment. On the other hand, the supervisory or veteran employee may continue to work without interruption while receiving treatment for a significant injury. His complaints are more likely to be genuine and confirmed by objective evidence, and they usually respond to proper treatment.

The individual who shifts from one job to another and has one or more previous compensation claims, may have a personality disorder which is reflected in various subjective or functional complaints; these are often exaggerated and may occasionally represent actual malingering. A few well directed questions may reveal pertinent information which may corroborate a suspected functional basis for his complaints. For example, other employees may have been involved in the same accident and, after sustaining similar types of injuries, have long since returned to work. All the injured are often treated by the same physician, particularly if he is associated with a Workmen's Compensation clinic which services that particular company.

Sometimes a patient makes an appointment for diagnosis and treatment several weeks or even several months after the injury, with a history of having received no treatment for it except at a hospital emergency room immediately after the accident. The doctor should discreetly inquire if the patient is about to make settlement with the insurance company, which is in all probability the real reason for his visit. Often the attorney wishes to learn the final status of his client prior to any negotiation of settlement. In these cases, the findings are ordinarily negative, but nevertheless a thorough examination should be performed to eliminate any possibility of residual disability. Usually such a patient is apprehensive and needs reassurance rather than treatment. He may fear recurrent permanent physical disability, or else the need of further medical care which he will have to pay for out of his own pocket after his case has been irrevocably settled. The physician should sit down and discuss the results of his examination with the patient so that he can proceed with a final disposition of the claim. If the physician is aware of the underlying reason for the patient's visit, it will facilitate his examination and management of the case.

It is helpful for the examining physician to know whether or not the patient is under the influence of any medication at the time of his examination, as this may influence test patterns. The patient should be questioned as to whether or not he has taken any medication on the day of examination and if so, type, dosage, and time. Although this is not the sole determining factor in his reactions, it may influence them to some extent. The patient will frequently give a vague answer to such questions, either not knowing what his doctor has prescribed or else not wishing to divulge its identity. If the patient has been taking medication over a long period of time, it is likely that he would have some idea as to what he is taking; if the patient is intelligent but professes ignorance, this should be considered in the final interpretation and evaluation.

EXAMINATION

The patient should be undressed sufficiently to permit a complete examination of the injured areas of the body, including comparison with uninjured extremities. In order to examine the lower back properly, all clothes and shoes should be removed, and the patient dressed in an examination garment which opens in the back; removal of clothes only to the belt line is inadequate for a diagnosis of low back disorders. The upper half of the torso should be exposed for a neck injury, to permit inspection for atrophy, scoliosis, kyphosis, and inspection of the dorsolumbar spine, any back deformity, surgical scars, etc., which may contribute to the symptomatology. If the injury is limited to a hand or foot, the entire limb should be exposed and examined to determine any pre-existing deformity or disease which would influence the alleged disability.

It may be helpful if the examiner observes the patient before she undresses to prepare for the examination; if she is seen when she enters the waiting room or while her history is being taken by the receptionist, for example, her dress or general appearance may offer a clue to her general make up and emotional pattern. Although it is well known that females will go to extremes to improve their appearance, it is questionable that an individual actually suffering from constant discomfort would devote much time and effort to personal appearance for the purpose of a defendant examination. On the other hand, some females obviously try to charm the doctor, hoping to favorably influence the examiner's report by personal appearance and attractiveness.

This attitude was illustrated by an attractive, middle-aged female who entered the office wearing a fancy hat pinned to a fashionable hair styling; in addition she was wearing long false eyelashes, and her eye shadow was beautifully done. During the preliminary history she whimpered as she told the receptionist how much persistent pain she had in her neck and back and recited her inability to tolerate any medicine, also her failure to respond to treatment. The receptionist complimented her on her excellent cosmetic preparation and her gorgeous hairdo and unusual hat. Having observed that the unusual head piece would be difficult to attach, the receptionist naïvely asked how the patient could do this while having so much pain and discomfort; the patient responded that it had required one and a half hours to get ready for her appointment.

During the examination the patient refused to take off her hat so that the doctor could inspect the head and neck, stating it was too complicated to re-attach it (which was true!). She repeated her complaints to the doctor, saying that nothing had helped, she just couldn't go on, and so forth. The doctor completed as much of the examination as possible with this restriction. In his conclusions the physician stated that the patient was extremely nervous and tense, but he could find no objective physical or x-ray findings to explain her continuing complaints.

This patient had been referred by her doctor for a consultation on behalf of the plaintiff. A short course of treatment was proposed by the orthopaedic consultant on a trial basis, but the patient did not wish to have any treatment which would mess up her hairdo. She did not want to return to his office for physical therapy, stating it was too much trouble to travel downtown from her home in the suburbs. Arrangements were then made for the physical therapy to be given in a suburban hospital near her home. Despite this convenience she kept only one appointment and then withdrew from care, indicating that the travel factor was not the true motivation for her lack of interest in therapy. The consultant was subpoenaed by the defense to testify in her case, after he had submitted his report, which stated these facts to the patient's attorney. The story of her initial appearance and failure to cooperate with proposed treatment was elicited from the doctor by the defense attorney. The jury, on which there were several women, was quite impressed with the doctor's description of the headpiece and his report regarding her hesitancy in removing it for the physical examination. They brought in a virtual defendant's verdict as she was given only three hundred dollars for her medical expenses.

Although the consultant was paid his usual expert witness fee by the defendant, he had difficulty in collecting his consultation fee from the patient. Only the strictest adherence to the assignment in his possession on the part of the plaintiff's attorney secured the payment. The angry patient and her husband blamed their defeat on the doctor, and initially refused to pay the bill until their attorney insisted.

A physical examination for the defendant should include all areas of the body in which the patient has had complaints. If the patient states he no longer has any difficulty with an area previously symptomatic, this region should still be examined as he may state he has additional symptoms in this area at a later date. Usually it is preferable to cover the asymptomatic areas by a quick systematic plan, then examine the symptomatic or disabling areas with thorough and undivided attention.

Occasionally a plaintiff's attorney insists upon being present during the examination on behalf of the defendant. The reason for such a request is not always clear: perhaps it is an effort to intimidate the examining physician and limit his questioning of the patient, or to secure a more favorable report because of the fear of later cross-examination by the attorney. Physicians who have established reputations for minute questioning of details regarding the accident with little time spent on the physical examination itself, are subjected to this form of harrassment more often. It would appear, however, that if the attorney had objected to the examination by such a physician, a simpler approach would have been to request submission of additional names of proposed examiners. The situation also varies according to jurisdictions; in New York City this apparently is a regular occurrence in the conduct of a defendant's examination. Often the defendant's physician is required to make the examination in the plaintiff attorney's office, a radical deviation in the practice of medicine which would not be acceptable to most doctors. Obviously, it would be difficult to conduct a complete examination in a non-medical setting without the usual physical facilities, instruments, x-rays apparatus, and other essential equipment.

In small communities where there is a closer liaison between the medical and legal professions, insistence upon the presence of the patient's attorney is a rare occurrence. In most large metropolitan areas, it is usually made by attorneys of lesser reputation with considerable free time. When conducting an examination with an attorney present, there should be a clear understanding that the lawyer may witness the examination but he is not to interfere or make comments during the procedure. If the patient is a female, the patient and the attorney should understand that there may be some disrobing required, and the patient should consent to whatever exposure is necessary in the presence of her attorney. With nervous patients, or those of limited education and memory, the attorney may be helpful by providing precise items in the history from his doctor's reports which had not yet been made available to the defendant; in some instances he may offer a copy of the report or copies of x-ray reports, all of which may be of considerable aid to the examiner.

Although the doctor may dictate some of his physical findings and the history as he proceeds with the examination, he definitely should not dictate his diagnosis and conclusions in the presence of the attorney. Usually the lawyer will make notes and should the doctor make any subsequent changes in his report, he may be cross-examined on this point and embarrassed on the witness stand.

Some attorneys may request that the treating physician be present for the defendant examination, with or without the attendance of the attorney. This was more common in the past, as today most physicians have learned to refuse such requests as an infringement upon their professional status and the mutual respect among physicians. The attending physician should not participate in such an examination except under extraordinary circumstances, as he is not an advocate and his principal function is to treat the patient. Although he should prepare all necessary reports, it is not his duty to build up the plaintiff's case for successful legal prosecution. When another doctor plans to witness the defendant examination, the appointment should be scheduled at a mutually convenient time which will permit the examination to be conducted without delay and without interference from other patients. However, the procedure is undignified and places both the examining and witnessing physicians in an embarrassing situation, which should be avoided.

This was exemplified a few years ago when the chief of surgery of a large suburban hospital witnessed an examination by the author at the request of the plaintiff's attorney. Although the physicians were not previously acquainted, they knew each other by reputation. The plaintiff's physician was very friendly and after witnessing the thorough examination made by the author, commented that his own examination was much less complete. Apparently he communicated his thoughts to the plaintiff's attorney as shortly thereafter the case was settled. It would appear that the tactic boomeranged in this particular case!

A. Physical Examination—General Notes

The orthopaedic examination should include general observations in addition to a detailed examination of the injured parts. The examiner should note facial expressions which reflect whether the patient is ill at ease, tense, apprehensive, or in obvious pain; he should observe difficulty in ascending, sitting, or lying on the examining table, gait disturbances such as a limp or drop-foot gait, and any other pertinent physical manifestations.

If the patient seems to be tense or the history indicates a possible anxiety condition, a blood pressure reading may be informative, as hypertension is a frequent cause of anxiety, especially if untreated. Often an accident victim receives excellent care for his orthopaedic injuries, but his blood pressure has never been taken even though his physician has prescribed tranquilizers and sedatives for nervousness, which is possibly due to elevated blood pressure. If the blood pressure is high, a brief chest examination may reveal cardiac murmurs or accentuated, metallic second aortic sounds associated with essential hypertension or other signs such as engorged veins, pulsating vessels in the neck, etc.

A brief examination of the ears, eyes, nose, mouth and throat may point to nystagmus, deviation of the protruding tongue, facial weakness or other findings; encrusted blood in the ears or scalp from a head injury may be observed if the examination is performed soon after the accident. Large or obese individuals should be weighed and their body build noted; a statement should be made whether their overweight status is chronic or recent. A recent gain in weight may indicate inactivity from enforced idleness as a result of the injury, whereas chronic obesity is often associated with hypertension or glandular dysfunction.

Notes should be made as the examination proceeds, preferably with a recording machine or dicated to a secretary. The doctor should not rely upon memory to write his report after the examination is completed, as the delay will undoubtedly result in omission or inaccuracy in some of the observations.

The doctor may wish to utilize outlines of an examination form or charts in which he may readily insert figures during his examination, such as blood pressure, leg length measurements, calf measurements, range of motion of the joints, and so forth (Figure 2). The use of such forms not only will expedite the writing down of basic information, but will facilitate a complete examination without omission. In addition the doctor can jot down his findings without dictating them in the presence of the patient, who may interject remarks objecting to negative observations of the examiner, particularly if this is a defendant examination.

A list of forms is appended which may serve as a useful outline, subject to the physician's own modifications. The forms include an outline of an examination for injury to the cervical spine, outline of interval reports to check on progress while under treatment, and outline of a final examination. The forms should not be utilized routinely without change, but they may form a basis for the complete examination and can be modified according to each individual patient. The type of occupation involved should also be noted, particularly when the patient is being returned to work after a prolonged absence. Other forms may be useful when there appears to be gross exaggeration of complaints; by using written forms, the physician can make observations

PHYSICAL EXAMINATION: Blood pressure_____/_____   ENT_____   H&L_____
                          Grip test Rt_____Lt_____ Rt handed_____ Lt. Handed_____

NECK MOTION: Rotation: Rt_____Lt_____
                          Lateral Flexion Rt_____Lt_____
                          Forward Flexion_____Extension_____

LEG LENGTH: Rt_____Lt_____   Reflexes:_____
                                              Sensation_____

CIRCUMFERENCE: Calves____" above malleoli Rt___Lt___ Arms___" above olecranon
                          Thighs____ """"""""""""""   Rt___Lt___ Forearms___ " below """"""

KNEE CIRCUMFERENCE: (MP) Rt_____Lt_____
KNEE MOTION: Rt_____Lt_____
ANKLE MOTION: Rt_____Lt_____

X-RAYS:

DIAGNOSIS:

RECOMMENDATIONS AND TREATMENT:
MEDICATION:

TREATMENT AND PROGRESS NOTES:

FIGURE 2. EXAMINATION FORM FOR NOTATIONS
OF MEASUREMENTS.

without calling the patient's attention to the notes being taken in his presence.

The following are suggested outlines for an orthopaedic examination of the cervical spine and lumbar spine and lower extremities. These forms include salient points in the examination which should be included in the report. As suggested, the examiner should use this only as a guide and supplement the form according to individual findings. In other words, it is not meant to be used as a "rubber stamp report," but should be modified or added to as the case demands.

Cervical Spine

"Moves the head and neck easily, with no evident distress. Biceps, triceps and radial reflexes are equal and normally active in both arms. Sensation, including pinprick and vibration sense, intact in both upper extremities. Circulation intact with symmetrical and normal skin temperature and color. Normal radial pulses in both arms. Shoulders are symmetrical and well developed, with a full range of overhead elevation, external and internal rotation and lateral abduction. No weakness of biceps, triceps or deltoid muscles against resistance. Performs a good trapezius shrug without difficulty or pain. Lateral cervical compression test causes no radicular pain to either upper extremity or shoulders. No tenderness or muscle spasm in the anterior, posterior or lateral cervical regions. No enlargement of the cervical lymph nodes; thyroid gland not enlarged or tender. Shoulder depression test negative.

Cervical motion: A) lateral flexion, right: Left:
                 B) forward flexion: Extension:
                 C) lateral rotation, right: Left:
"Grip testing, Jamar Dynanometer, right: Repeat: right:
                                       left: left:
Right-handed_____ Left-handed _____

"Patient moves head and neck easily during the ENT examination as constrasted to direct observation during measurement of range of motion."

Lumbar Spine

"Stand erect with pelvis and shoulders level; satisfactory posture. Bends forward with fingertips _____ inches from touching the floor. Good range of lateral flexion and backward extension without discomfort or restriction. With forward flexion, there is rounding and reversal of the lumbar curve, indicating lack of any muscle spasm in this area. No tenderness or muscle spasm in the dorsal, lumbar or gluteal regions. No increased sensitivity over the gluteal portion of the sciatic nerve. No tenderness about the trochanteric regions of the hips. Full range of motion in both hips, including abduction and adduction, flexion, extension, and internal-external rotation. Full flexion and extension of knees with good muscle power without pain or restriction.

"Leg length _____ inches on the right and _____ inches left; calf circumference measured at _____ inches above the medial malleolus is _____ inches on the right and _____ inches on the left. Thigh circumference measured at _____ inches from the medial malleolus is _____ inches on the right and _____ inches on the left. Calves and thighs symmetrical, measured at comparative distances from the medial malleoli.

Knee jerks and ankle jerks are equal and normally active. Sensation, including pinprick and vibration sense intact in both lower extremities. The skin temperature and color are symmetrical. No swelling of the ankles. Has good power of toe flexion-extension with no weakness demonstrated; able to walk on toes and heels well. Straight leg-raising accomplished to _____ degrees without difficulty. Lasègue, Naffziger and Patrick tests negative bilaterally. Yeoman hip hyperextension test negative bilaterally. Patient is able to turn over on the examining table without difficulty and also gets up and down from the table without any obvious difficulty. Walks with normal gait.

"With the patient lying face down in the prone position, knees flexed 90 degrees, patient complains of definite discomfort in the _____ area as a result of toe flexion and extension (no anatomical association between the maneuver performed and the alleged increased discomfort). Hyperextends the mid and upper back against gravity without difficulty."

Examination of Lower Extremities

"Stands with pelvis level. Walks with normal gait. Walks well on toes and heels, no asymmetry of the lower extremities. No swelling of the ankles. Popliteal spaces are normal, no masses, no swelling, no tenderness. Has a full range of motion in both knees from 0 to _____ degrees. Leg lengths equal, measured from the anterior superior iliac spine to the inferior margin of the medial malleoli, _____ inches left and right.

"Mid-patellar circumference of the knees right and left _____ inches; circumference of calves measured _____ inches above the medial malleoli _____ inches; thighs measured _____ inches above the medial malleoli, right and left _____ inches. Knee jerks and ankle jerks are equal and normally active. Sensation, including pin prick and vibration sense, intact. Pulsations in posterior tibial and anterior dorsalis pedis vessels are normal. Has a full range of motion in both hips, including abduction and adduction, flexion, extension, internal and external rotation. No crepitus with hip motion. No pain with motion. Lasègue, Patrick and Leguerre tests negative for both hips. Good muscle strength in both lower extremities, including quadriceps, hamstrings, and calf muscles."

The following is a brief outline of an examination of ears, nose, and throat, neurological signs, and heart and lungs, in addition to the procedures in the orthopaedic examination. A more detailed neurological examination should be performed by a neurologist or a neurosurgeon if indicated.

ENT

"Pupils are equal and react to light and accommodation. Tongue protrudes in the midline. No tremor of tongue. No facial weakness. Wrinkles forehead easily. Jaw opening is symmetrical. No bleeding or other discharge from ears, nose, mouth or throat. No nystagmus. No scars of recent injury."

Neurological

"Romberg test negative. Finger-to-nose test negative. Good coordination. No tremor of hands. Normal gait. Performs alternating movements of hands well (no adiadochokinesis).

Chest

"Heart—normal rate and rhythm; no murmurs. Lungs are clear and resonant throughout. Symmetrical chest expansion of _____ inches or _____ cm with no pain with deep inspiration. No friction fremitus; no rales."

Outlines of tests performed to determine validity of complaints may be prepared in advance and used when dictating the examination in the presence of the patient. This will insure that the pertinent data are included in the examination report, as the doctor may forget to include them if he defers the dictation until after the examination is concluded. He may be rushed with other patients, phone calls, etc., but with such a form he can make a quick notation and insert it in the chart for inclusion in his report.

Suggested Tests

1. Patient states he is quite tender when palpated in the _____ area, but with attention diverted and simultaneous palpation elsewhere and patient engaged in conversation, the identical area is again palpated with firmer pressure and no pain reaction elicited. This would indicate inconsistency, for had the area actually been tender, the pain would have been elicited whether or not the patient's attention was focused on the area (such as when twisting an acutely sprained ankle).

2. With patient standing in the erect position, arms behind him, he/she claims increased discomfort pointing to the back of the neck and across the shoulders, as a result of the physician's gripping the mid-arms and squeezing the mid-arms in this position (no anatomical association).

3. With the patient erect, elbows flexed 90 degrees, patient is asked to clench his hands into a tight fist with the examiner squeezing his hands in this position; patient alleges discomfort in the back of his neck as a result of this maneuver (no anatomical association).

4. A good test for the "insurance claim malingerer" with backache: the patient lies face down with legs flexed 90 degrees at the knees. If he complains of pain in the back when the toes

are flexed or extended against resistance in this position, then his "back problem" should be seriously questioned. Muscles activating the toes originate below the knee, and could not anatomically cause pain in the pelvic or lumbar areas. Some "performers" scream loudly with alleged pain and try to crawl off the examining table, then claim persistent discomfort for hours after this simple test.

B. Extremities

Comparative measurements should be made of the length and girth of the upper or lower extremities where indicated, using specific reference points for recording circumference, such as 8 to 10 inches from the medial malleolus to the calves, 20 to 25 inches from the medial malleolus or 10 to 11 inches downward from the anterior inferior iliac spine for circumference of the thighs, infrapatellar, midpatellar, and suprapatellar circumferences of the knees, etc. In the upper extremities, the circumferences of the mid-arms and forearms may be measured at points 4 to 5 inches above and below the olecranon process. This gives definite information regarding muscular atrophy, swelling, edema of the ankles, and so forth. If a patient states he has had repeated swelling of the affected parts, such as the foot and ankle, measurements are of value in corroborating this complaint. Absence of atrophy would reflect active use of the extremity; this observation is important if the patient claims great discomfort and persistent disability. Bony land-marks are used to measure leg length.

Physicians vary in their interpretations of mild degrees of leg length discrepancies. Some physicians believe that any shortening up to ½ inch is within normal limits, but most agree that more than ¼ inch should be considered significant. Studies have indicated that 12 per cent of individuals have irregular growth of the lower extremities, resulting in leg length discrepancies of up to ¼ inch, sometimes slightly more, without any history of disease or injury. This may account for a minor difference in leg length with no history of fracture, poliomyelitis, or neurological disorder. Discrepancies in leg length can cause backache from a secondary tilting of the pelvis and unbalanced mechanics of the lower back.

A goniometer is used to measure range of motion of peripheral joints, such as elbow, wrist and knee. Range of motion of joints should be recorded, using the standard nomenclature recommended by the American Academy of Orthopaedic Surgeons, which will avoid confusion in comparative evaluations by other physicians. Specific degrees of motion should be recorded whenever possible, using comparative charts for the fingers or wrists so that the reader may note at a glance any differences between the injured and uninjured areas.

The following chart may serve as a helpful form on which to record detailed and comparative data for hand and arm evaluation. This form provides a handy method of jotting down ranges of motion in the elbows, wrists, and hands, circumference measurements, and grip testing results. Such a notation permits ready comparison of the uninjured and injured sides which is particularly useful for the small finger joints. Loss of motion is easily observed when compared side by side (Figure 3).

C. Grip Testing

Weakness of the hands and forearms should be recorded by grip testing, using a scientific apparatus such as the Jamar Dynamometer, and repeating the readings to check their accuracy or to test for malingering. (Figure 4).

The grip should be accurately tested in all injuries involving the upper extremities or the cervical spine, in order to detect any motor weakness of the extremities resulting from a direct injury to the extremity, such as a fracture, or from paralysis of the motor nerves and muscles of the upper extremity, such as injury to the nerve roots which emerge from the cervical spine. When scientifically tested, the results can be informative; they are of significant value if they are consistent with other positive physical findings such as a measurable atrophy of the extremities, linear or angular deformities of the forearm, wrist, or digits due to fracture, partial ankylosis or limited motion of the shoulder, elbow, wrist, or fingers, etc. Usually the grip is greater in the dominant hand of the individual, i.e. the right hand of a right-handed person. This is more consistently noted in right-handed

HAND & ARM EVALUATION

PATIENT: _____

Date _____

Injured Hand R   L

Dominant Hand R   L

ARM:	RIGHT	LEFT
Circumference		
(___ inches from olecranon)		

ELBOW:	RIGHT	LEFT
Flexion		
Extension		

FOREARM:	RIGHT	LEFT
Pronation		
Supination		
Circumference		
(___ inches above radial styloid)		

WRIST:	RIGHT	LEFT
Volar Flexion		
Dorsiflexion		
Ulnar Deviation		
Radial Deviation		
Circumference		
(at radial styloid)		

HAND GRIP (Jamar Dynamometer)	RIGHT (lbs.)	LEFT (lbs.)
1		
2		
3		
4		

HAND MOTION

		Thumb - 1st		Index - 2nd		Middle - 3rd		Ring - 4th		Little - 5th	
		R	L	R	L	R	L	R	L	R	L
A. Metacarpo-Phalangeal Joint	Flexion										
	Extension										
B. Proximal Interphalangeal Joint	Flexion										
	Extension										
C. Distal Interphalangeal Joint	Flexion										
	Extension										
D. Approximation of finger to palm (loss)											

FIGURE 3. HAND AND ARM EVALUATION.

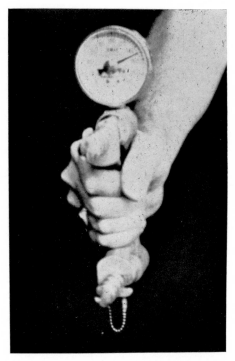

FIGURE 4. JAMAR DYNAMOMETER.

individuals, as many left-handed individuals are somewhat am-
bidextrous in the use of their upper extremities and often have
an equal grip bilaterally.

Grip also varies according to sex, age, occupation and body
build. Most adult males can grip above 50 pounds with the
Jamar grip tester, with the exception of the aged and infirm.
Although some females may also exert such a grip, most sedentary
types have a grip of 25 to 50 pounds on the dominant side. There
is usually no greater than a 20 to 25 per cent difference between
the dominant and subordinate hand.

The use of an accurate grip measurement is significant not
only for diagnosis, but also for the information needed to assist
the proper placement of the employee for work after an injury
involving the hand or upper extremity. The employee can be
given a job that he can perform without detriment to his health

as well as with satisfactory results for his employer. Manual grip testing is unsatisfactory as it is a subjective measurement which gives no basis for either comparative measurement or later reference to evaluate progress. However, manual testing can be helpful in detecting malingering and the lack of full voluntary effort; if the examiner places one hand on the forearm and grips the patient's hand with the other, the voluntary contractures of the forearm muscles can be palpated, thereby detecting the amount of effort exerted.

The results of grip testing should be consistent after a short rest period. Using the Jamar adjustable dynamometer, repeat tests can be performed after a short interval of rest. There should be no more than a 10 per cent deviation on retest. However, where there is definite doubt as to the cooperation of the patient, a complete test can be performed in the following fashion: the grip test is first carried out in the usual manner, and results recorded for all grip sizes available on the dynamometer. There is an optimum opening at which the patient is able to grip with more force than any other. After a lapse of five minutes or more, during which time the remainder of the physical examination can be conducted, the test is repeated and again recorded. The results should not vary more than 10 per cent, regardless of the size of the opening. If there has been less than maximum effort exerted, the variation in reading may be as great at 100 per cent. In some cases, the examiner may wish to permit the subject to see the dial during the first test, so that he will be aware of the reading in both hands; after a five-minute lapse, have the subject repeat the test without seeing the dial. If he is attempting to simulate a voluntarily controlled first test, it is unlikely that he will be able to do so within the 10 per cent range. Malingering can thus be detected in a valid manner by objective and scientific testing that can be accurately described in testimony, if required.[23]

D. Cervical Spine

Examination of the cervical spine should include an estimate or measurement of range of motion, including lateral rotation, lateral flexion, forward flexion and hyperextension; this can be performed fairly accurately with the Cervigon apparatus. The Cervigon apparatus is composed of two parts: one is a flat protractor scale with a chin piece that measures lateral rotation to either side; the other is a crownlike device with two protractor scales, one to measure lateral tilt to either side and the other for an estimate of flexion and extension motions. There are also other types of apparatus on the market (e.g. a fluid goniometer) which are designed to estimate ranges of cervical motion; the examiner should select the device of his choice, then use it regularly in his practice (Figure 5).

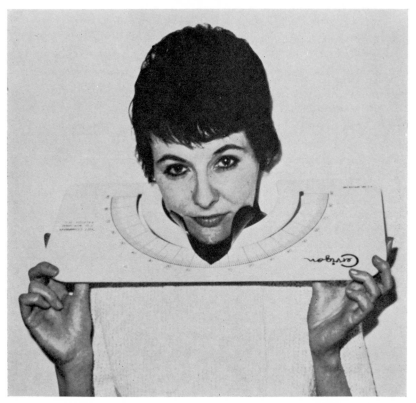

FIGURE 5. MEASUREMENT OF RANGE OF MOTION OF CERVICAL SPINE, (USING THE CERVIGON APPARATUS).
   A. Lateral rotation.

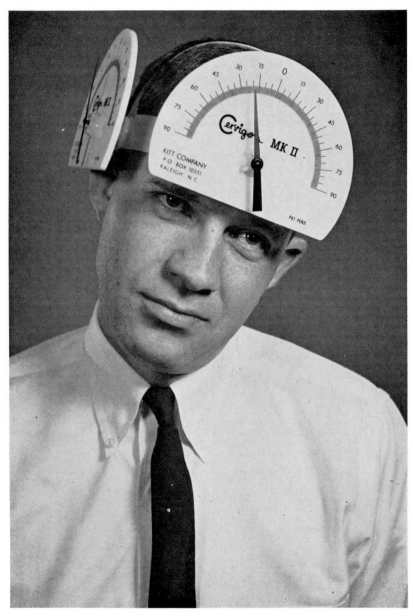

B. Left lateral tilt or flexion.

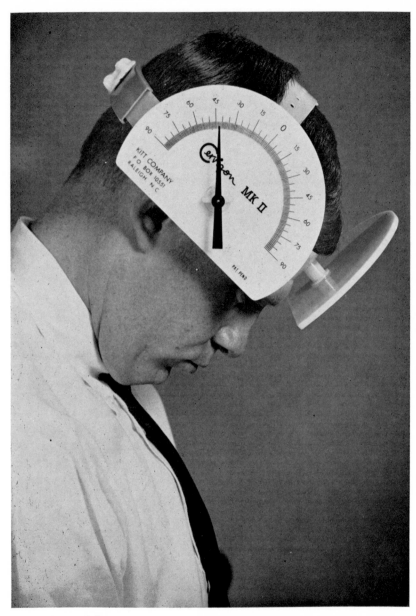

C. Forward flexion.

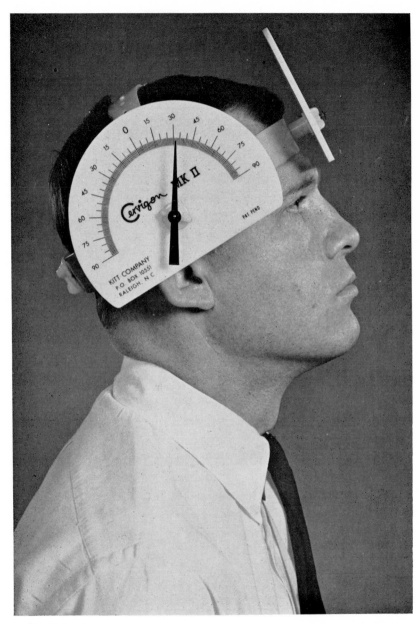

D. Extension.

A neurological examination of the upper extremities is necessary after a cervical injury; the biceps, triceps, and radial reflexes and sensation including vibratory sense should be tested and recorded. The sensory testing should be done with a rotating pinwheel and/or spring-loaded tension pin (i.e. Crowe anesthesiometer: Richards and Co.); a good tuning fork (C-128) is helpful in evaluating vibratory sensation. If there is stocking or glove type of hypesthesia of the lower or upper extremity, often involving half of the trunk on the same side, the examiner should suspect a significant neurotic or functional element rather than organic injury. However, organic hypesthesia is sometimes obscured by a functional overlay with an overflow of the hypesthesia to non-involved areas. Hypesthesia following definite anatomical patterns may indicate a cervical or lumbar disc syndrome. Muscular atrophy and weakness of specific muscles against resistance should be noted and tests for radiculitis such as lateral arm traction and lateral cervical compression performed and recorded.

Localized tenderness and muscle spasm should be carefully observed and evaluated by retesting as frequently there is a large subjective or voluntary component, or the patient may involuntarily tighten his musculature from apprehension of anticipated pain. Visual and palpable detection of muscle spasm may be difficult on a purely objective basis, but an experienced examiner can make a fairly accurate determination. Involuntary muscle spasm persists throughout the examination but where there is voluntary control, the spasm is present only as the area is directly examined, being relaxed when attention is diverted from the specific area. If the patient has pain with certain motions of the neck and shoulders, it should be evaluated according to anatomical considerations of stretching and relaxation as the head is turned to one side or the other. Where the statements are at variance with the known anatomical pattern, corroborative evidence should be secured by further testing.

E. Lower Extremities

Examination of the lower extremities should include observations of gait patterns, limb length, and distribution of weight bearing, noting any tendency to shift weight away from the injured area. Abrasions, contusions and lacerations should be described, their approximate size, severity, and apparent relationship to the accident being indicated wherever possible. Ranges of motion in the hips, knees, and ankles should be measured and reported in detail if there is any impairment of joint function. Joint effusions should be noted and reported with comparative measurements of the knees or ankles. The examiner should check for joint and ligamentous instability, crepitus, cysts, evidences of traumatic tendinitis, circulatory problems and nerve deficit.

Joint effusion is sometimes overlooked when the extremity is examined in the reclining position; a small effusion may be detected only with the patient in the erect position, allowing gravitation and accumulation of the excessive joint fluid. Thus, a suprapatellar bursa will bulge in the erect position, indicating an easily recognized joint effusion which otherwise is dispersed when the patient lies on the examining table. (However, occasionally the reverse is true.) Comparative measurements of the knees made in the erect position at the suprapatellar level may reveal soft tissue redundancy and thickening which are not apparent with the patient lying on his back. This is especially true in obese individuals or with abnormally relaxed skin and subcutaneous tissues.[15,17]

F. Back—Diagnostic Tests

The back should first be examined with the patient in the upright position without shoes, and particular attention be given to any scoliosis, kyphosis, or lordosis; the examiner should also observe for accentuation of lateral curves with the back flexed and see whether the overall pattern compensates for the scoliotic curve (a carpenter's plumb bob is excellent for this). The amount of forward flexion should be recorded, measuring the distance of the fingertips to the floor and noting also disappearance or flattening of the normal lordotic curve with acute flexion of the lumbar spine; this occurs in the absence of muscle spasm, but will not occur if true muscle spasm is present (Figure 6).

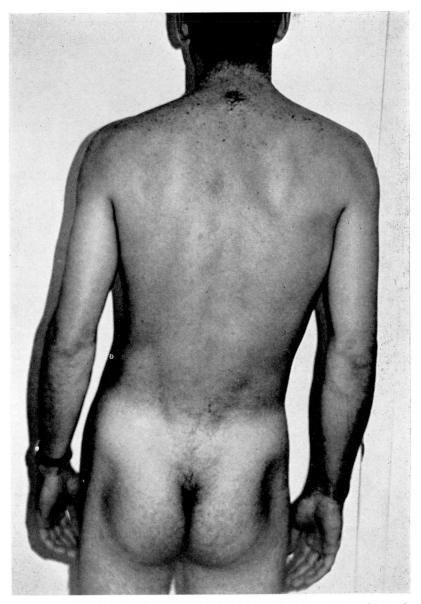

FIGURE 6. EXAMINATION OF THE BACK: Objective Signs of Muscle
    Spasm.
    A. Pelvic tilt to the right: trunk shifted to the right; result of muscle
        spasm.

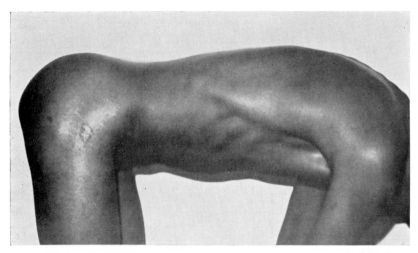

B. Persistence of lumbar curvature in flexion with no reversal of lordosis; true muscle spasm present.

Range of right and left lateral flexion and torsion with the hips flexed should be noted, together with any pain produced by these motions; usually pain occurs on the ipsilateral side with a disc protrusion (from compression of the herniated disc against the emerging nerve roots), and on the contralateral side with a muscle or ligamentous strain (stretching of the injured ligament). Forward flexion usually aggravates disc pain, whereas backward extension usually increases the pain resulting from lumbosacral muscle strain.

The location of tenderness should be noted carefully; when the patient alleges tenderness over a bony area as the mid or lower sacrum, where ligamentous strains cannot occur, it may indicate a functional, non-organic etiology. The presence of a herniated fat pad can be detected by careful palpation in the lumbar and upper gluteal areas, preferably with the back flexed; a tender palpable fat pad may result from a severe ligamentous strain or localized trauma from an accident.

Patients who claim inability to bend forward more than a few degrees in the erect position should be carefully observed when dressing or sitting, and also tested by back flexion while sitting on the examining table. With the knees fully extended, they are asked to sit up and try to touch their toes, simulating the same maneuver as in the standing position when bending to touch their toes. A patient who is not malingering or exaggerating will demonstrate the identical range of motion whether standing or sitting on the table, whereas the claims-conscious individual will flex his back appreciably better from the sitting position. Observation of the patient bending down to put on his shoes or getting on and off the examining or x-ray table will also give corroborative evidence. The alert physician may sometimes observe the allegedly disabled patient when he leaves the office or walks down the corridor, to note any differences in gait and behavior patterns when not under direct observation. During the examination the patient's gestures and behavior will often give a clue to an experienced observer, indicating neurotic or anxiety manifestations, exaggeration, or malingering.

Straight leg raising, Lasègue, Naffziger, Laguerre, Patrick, Yeoman's hip hyperextension tests, Gaenslen's test and Ober's test should be performed. Observations should be made regarding tight hamstring muscles or contractures which often limit back motion (Figure 7).[13,16,18,20]

When the patient moves his knees, head and neck, or the back in a jerky, cogwheel fashion, it is usually a sign of voluntary control with an associated nervous factor. This is often observed when he is coming up from a flexed position of the lumbar spine, straightening up slowly with jerky and apparently painful movements.[11]

Functional Manifestations of the Lower Back

A functional basis of continued complaints can be determined with a tuning fork by testing each side of a single spinous process, testing first on one side, then the opposite side. If sensation is present in one half and not in the other, this is obviously a functional manifestation, as vibration is transmitted through the entire bony process.

A patient who complains about pain in one leg may become confused when he is rapidly turned over, from front to back or back to front; when asked to point to the painful leg, he may point to the wrong one, which certainly should not occur if he is having real pain in that leg.

The evaluation of back motion is sometimes difficult as patients frequently are apprehensive and hold themselves volun-

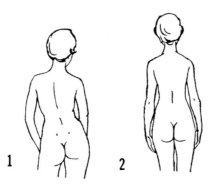

FIGURE 7. EXAMINATION OF THE BACK:
    A. OBSERVATIONS: the patient should have minimal protective covering during the examination so that all joints, the spine and muscles can be clearly observed during the tests. Look for body list, level shoulders, pelvic tilt, scoliosis:
    1. Pelvic tilt to the left; body list to the left.
    2. Shoulders and pelvis level; no scoliosis.

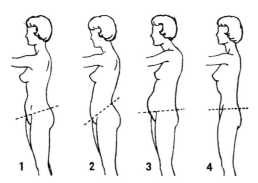

    B. STANDING POSTURE:
    1. Normal.
    2. Increased lumbar lordosis.
    3. Lordosis, prominent abdomen, obese.
    4. Slender.

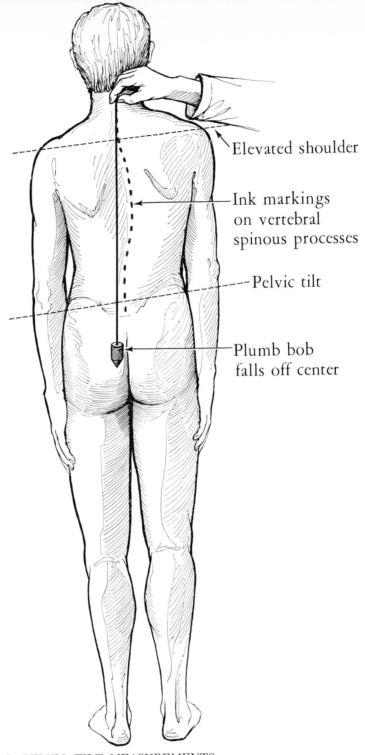

Elevated shoulder

Ink markings
on vertebral
spinous processes

Pelvic tilt

Plumb bob
falls off center

C. PELVIC TILT MEASUREMENTS:

1. Examine the patient from front and rear while standing, to determine pelvic tilt. Pelvic tilt from the rear is sometimes more easily observed by placing an ink dot in the center of each dimple or depression on either side of L-3 and L-4.

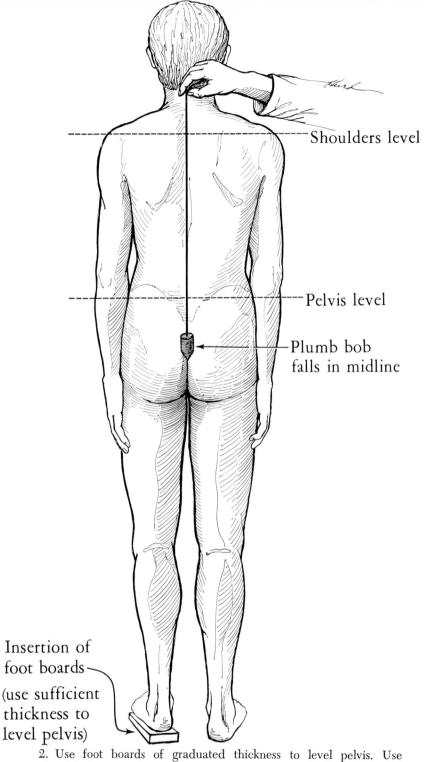

Shoulders level

Pelvis level

Plumb bob
falls in midline

Insertion of
foot boards
(use sufficient
thickness to
level pelvis)

2. Use foot boards of graduated thickness to level pelvis. Use plumb bob to test for compensation of lateral curves. Lumbar strain results from pelvic tilt without compensatory shoe corrections.

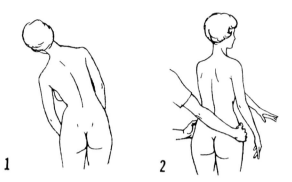

1   2

D. LATERAL FLEXION AND TORSION IN STANDING POSI-
   TION: Observe for limitation of motion to either side, and pain
   produced with motion toward pain side, or away from pain side.
   With pelvis tilted to one side, pain produced on same side by downward and lateral compression is typical of disc protrusion and nerve
   root irritation. Pain produced on opposite side by lateral flexion
   is more often associated with lumbar strain.
   1. Tilting truck to left or right, with or without pain.
   2. Twisting trunk with or without pain.

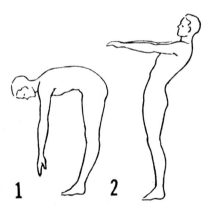

1   2

E. FLEXION AND EXTENSION MOVEMENTS: Note rounding and
   reversal of lumbar lordotic curve in flexed position. Measure distance
   of fingertips from floor. Note range of backward extension. Note
   pain associated with either flexion or extension motions.
   1. Flexion.
   2. Extension.

tarily tense, often refusing to exhibit any forward flexion whatsoever, particularly in the standing position. However, when sitting on the examining table with legs completely stretched out and knees at 180 degrees, the patient may then be able to flex his back forward well past 90 degrees, with fingertips approaching toes, indicating a considerable amount of back flexion

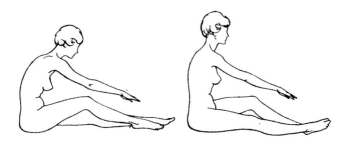

1

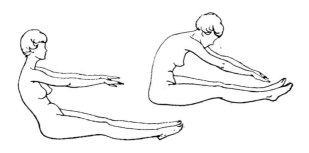

2

Flexion

F. HAMSTRING CONTRACTURES—SITTING TESTS:

1. Flexion with knees flexed: to determine contracture of hamstring muscles on either side, which could inhibit full forward flexion of lumbar spine.

2. Flexion in sitting position with knees extended, performed to corroborate range of motion observed in erect position. Positive for lumbar rigidity, sciatic scoliosis, muscle spasm and vertebral ankylosis. Normal if able to touch toes or ankles.

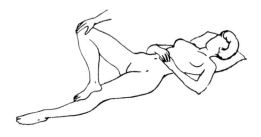

1

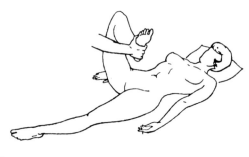

2

G. TESTS FOR HIP JOINT AND SACRO-ILIAC DISEASE:
   1. Crossing leg: Fabere-Patrick's test (heel placed on opposite knee
   and then leg and knee are forced to table). Positive for localizing
   right or left hip joint disease or sacro-iliac pain.
   2. Laguerre's test: external rotation of hip in abduction with knee
   flexed. If positive, similar to Fabere-Patrick test.

which he had not previously demonstrated in the erect position.

   Another common problem is a limp or bizarre gait pattern
which is inconsistent with the negative physical examination.
The patient should be observed both inside and outside the
examination room. If it is a true gait defect, it will persist unchanged whether or not the patient realizes he is being observed.

   The following observations will aid the examiner in dis-
tinguishing between organic and functional manifestations, or
malingering:

   1. Patient reports pain caused by straight leg raising while

lying down, then no pain when he is in the sitting position and the same maneuver is performed.

2. There are complaints of pain with hip flexion with the knees bent; however, this position does not stretch, but relieves the tension on the muscles, ligaments and nerves, and should not be painful.

3. In the absence of any hip disease, patient complains of pain on rotation of the hips, complaining of more pain than with straight leg raising.

4. Patient's complaint of pain with very light fingertip or skin type pressure over the back usually is a sign of non-organic disease; with a herniated disc, there is pain only with firm pressure over the involved interspace or well localized over the area of an acute ligamentous strain.

5. Pain is reported with light touch over bony prominences such as the mid sacrum; this is not consistent with ligamentous or muscular injury or herniated disc pathology. Pain that does not follow a consistent pattern according to known neuromuscular pathways may be questioned; pain arising at S-1 usually radiates behind the calf, and pain from L-4 nerve roots would go to the anterior thigh or anterior medial aspect of the leg.

6. Vague weakness of the extremity with no specific weakness

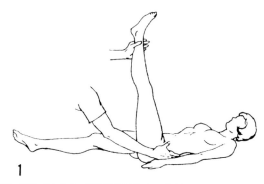

1

H. LYING ON BACK (SUPINE) TESTS:
   1. Straight leg raising test with patient lying on back. Normal straight leg raising varies from 75 to 90 degrees, depending upon muscular development, age, previous exercise patterns.

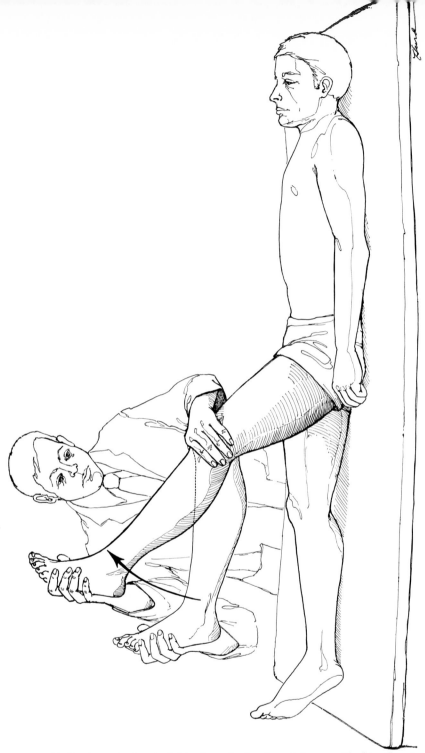

2. Lasègue test—straightening of the flexed knee with hip flexed produces additional stretch on sciatic nerve and causes pain along nerve pathways with sciatic nerve neuritis.

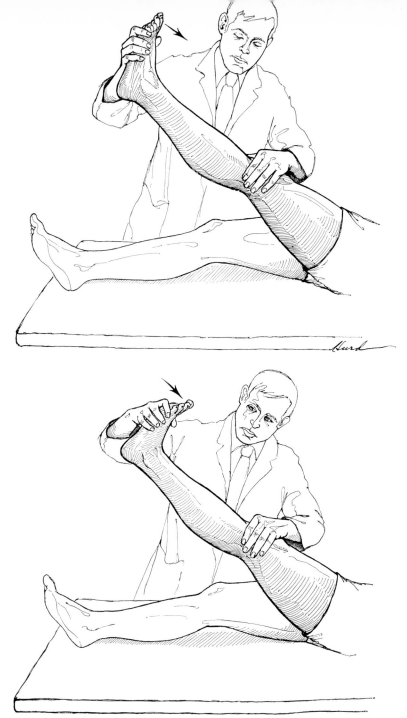

3. Naffziger test—with knee extended, hip flexed, ankle is forcibly
dorsiflexed, placing a final stretch on sciatic nerve root components.
Positive if pain is evidenced along nerve pathway, indicating minimal
to mild sciatic neuritis.

Lumbosacral spine disease is indicated when pain is observed in this
area as stretching legs begins to cause spinal movement.

should also be questioned, such as toe flexion or extension with no evidence of a massive disc protrusion.

7. Sensory losses that follow no known organic pathways, usually of the stocking or glove type, are in the same category.

8. Vague pains that are said to radiate from the low back up to the head, or from the head and neck down to the low back, are usually not organic in nature.[11]

In conducting his physical examination, the examiner must be careful that he does not reveal to the patient, either by word or facial expression, how he expects the patient to answer in response to his examining maneuvers. For example, in testing pinprick, he should not say, "You feel that, don't you?" or, "That is sharp, isn't it?" Rather, he should ask what the patient feels. A patient who has been examined more than once, or has been repeatedly examined by his own physician, may become knowledgeable and reply with the anticipated answer to a defendant examiner's questions, especially if asked in a suggestive manner. In evaluating litigation cases involving hysteria, malingering, or emotional disturbances, this can be an important factor.

Organic disease of the lower back can be diagnosed in most cases by a careful physical examination without the need of pantopaque myelography, but occasionally an electromyogram (neuro-muscular testing) may be indicated to add an objective basis to the clinical findings. This is a relatively benign test as compared to a myelogram and does not require hospitalization. However, the interpretation of the electromyogram is based on the experience and knowledge of the physiatrist conducting the examination and this subjective factor must also be weighed in evaluating the EMG report.

Aids to Differential Diagnosis of Acute Low Back Syndrome

In establishing a sound diagnosis for low back pains; the physician can avail himself of certain established guidelines as follows:

HERNIATED INTERVERTEBRAL DISC:

1. Pain begins immediately or within a few hours of injury in the lumbosacral area, then gradually spreads and becomes sciatic pain.

2. Pain is accentuated by forward bending, coughing, sneezing or any straining movement. Pain particularly restricts forward bending. Pain is accentuated by lateral compression towards the affected side.

3. Usually many attacks occur with spontaneous remissions, but they become gradually more intense and longer in duration.

4. Reproduction of sciatic pain with straight leg raising is a good clue.

5. If pressure or percussion over lumbar paravertebral area causes sciatic pain, a protruding disc is indicated.

6. Flexion of head and neck increases tension on extradural nerves in spinal canal.

7. Atrophy of leg muscles may be observed over some length of time.

8. Weakness of dorsiflexion of large toe and inability to walk on heels indicate 5th lumbar root involvement by 4th lumbar disc protrusion.

9. Inability to walk on toes because of calf muscle paresis and weakness of flexion of great toe, indicates 1st sacral root involvement by 5th lumbar disc protrusion.

10. In severe cases marked muscle spasm with spastic scoliosis, pelvic tilt and listing trunk may be observed.

11. Sensory signs are noted in 80 per cent of patients.

12. Reflexes of the ankle and the knee are reduced, respectively, when the 1st sacral and the 4th lumbar nerve roots are involved.

LOW BACK MUSCLE STRAIN:

1. Hemorrhage or subfacial hematoma is sometimes visible.

2. Muscle spasm can actually be seen or felt.

3. Localized tenderness is determined in prone position or with patient sitting on heels with back fully flexed (bent over knees).

4. If the spasm is severe enough, there may be some sciatic radiation, but ordinarily lack of radiation will indicate muscle strain only.

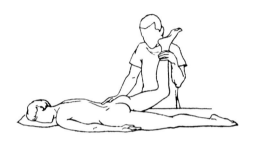

1

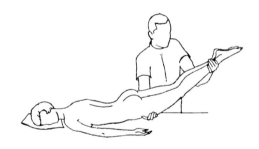

2

I. LYING ON FACE (PRONE) TESTS:

1. Hip Hyperextension test (Yeoman's): Raise whole leg with flexed knee and pelvis stabilized. This is positive for sacroiliac or lumbosacral strain when pain occurs on side of lesion, right or left, as force of hyperextension is transferred to the affected joint.

2. If Yeoman's test is found negative, then physician hyperextends both legs together. If pain is observed in lumbar spine or lower thoracic spine upon hyperextension of one or both legs, it may indicate arthritic changes or minimal strain.

5. Occasionally spasm in the legs is more clearly observed when the patient is undressed, if he is asked to walk a few steps.

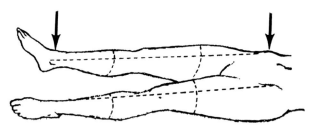

J. MEASUREMENTS:

1. Measure comparative leg lengths with patient supine (from medial malleolus to anterior iliac spine). Discrepancies exceeding ⅛ inch are significant and represent a frequent and often overlooked cause of low back strain.

2. Measure circumference of each thigh at mid point (measure 20 to 25 inches above medial malleolus depending on leg length).

3. Measure circumference of each calf at largest point, equidistant from medial malleolus. Diminution of ¼ inch or more may indicate muscle atrophy often associated with chronic or recurrent disc protrusions and sciatica.

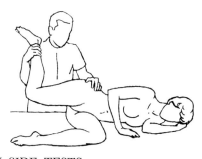

K. LYING ON SIDE TESTS.

1. Ober's test: Flex knee and fully extend the hip with opposite hip flexed, then allow the leg, knee and thigh to drop toward the table. This is positive for contracted tensor fasciae latae if the flexed knee does not drop to the table momentarily; present after poliomyelitis, hip joint disease, etc.

2. Compress pelvis with hands. Sacroiliac localization if pain is caused in either sacroiliac joint upon compression.

Movement is free during part of the range of motion but suddenly freezes, due to spasm which can be seen and felt.

6. Limitation and pain with back motion is observed especially upon hyperextension and lateral flexion away from the injured side.

7. Positive Yeoman hip hyperextension test indicates lumbosacral muscle strain.

X-RAYS

Roentgenographic examination is an important part of a medico-legal examination, both for positive and negative values. Whenever in doubt, the physician should recommend or take x-rays of the affected areas, using opposite extremities for comparison in doubtful studies. If the patient refuses to have x-rays taken as recommended, this reaction should be recorded in his medical record as a protection to the examining or treating physician.

The experienced orthopaedist will repeat x-rays after injuries to the rib cage, pelvis, hips, wrist, or other areas, whenever subjective complaints continue despite initially negative x-rays, as he realizes undisplaced fractures may not be apparent on x-rays made within the first two weeks (Figure 8). X-rays may be omitted in areas which have not been severely injured, but even negative x-rays are of considerable value when the case comes to trial, or if the patient continues to complain in the same area. In the latter case the x-rays may have to be repeated, even though they were initially negative, to establish firmly the diagnosis and prognosis.

If the x-rays were reported as negative but the patient continues to complain several months or years later, a physician examining for the defendant may repeat the x-rays to be sure a lesion was not overlooked or to identify any subsequent development. Repeatedly negative x-rays also bolster a diagnosis of non-organic basis for the patient's continued complaints, although soft tissue injuries are not excluded as they are not demonstrable by x-ray.

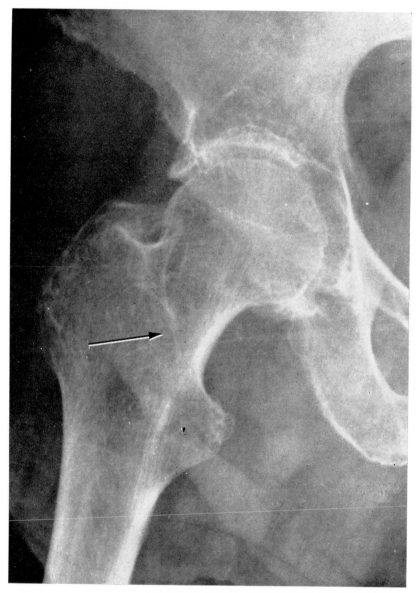

FIGURE 8. FRACTURE OF NECK OF FEMUR, NOT VISIBLE ON
INITIAL X-RAYS.
  A. Patient complained of pain in right hip, especially with rotation;
     local tenderness over right side of pelvis. Fracture of neck of femur
     suspected; Buck's extension traction applied to right leg. No fracture
     line visible on multiple views taken on admission.

If the examination is performed for a specific evaluation and prognosis, x-rays are important to lend weight to the conclusions. An excessive number of x-rays may be taken, but they are necessary to support the diagnosis and to protect the physician from a malpractice claim. A lay jury or judge often considers the examination incomplete without pertinent x-rays. The patients themselves frequently share this opinion, often attaching unwarranted importance to radiological examination. The defendant insurance company usually considers the financial investment for x-rays of minor importance in a complete examination, as negative x-rays are usually to their advantage and help the defending

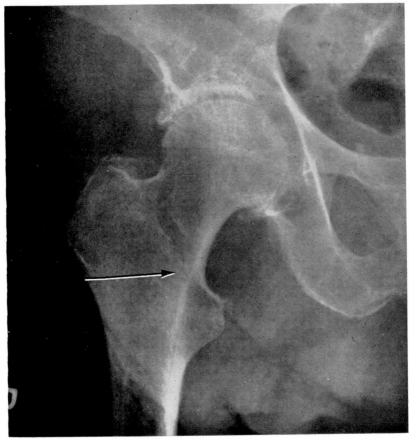

8. B. Eleven days after injury.

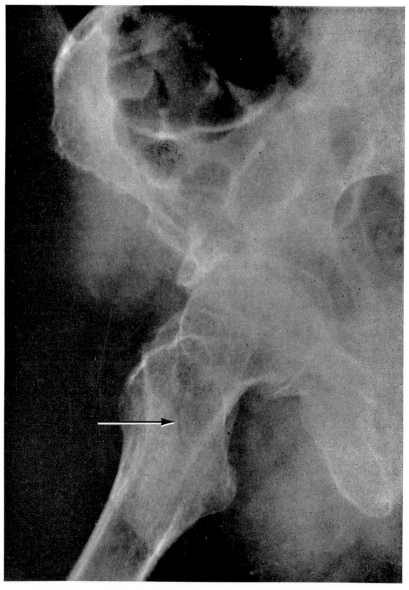

C. X-rays taken eleven days after admission. Decalcification along fracture line reveals undisplaced fracture of femoral neck in AP and lateral views. Four Knowles pins inserted with good result.

attorney. However, some patients object to proposed x-rays because of the extensive publicity regarding dangers of excessive radiation; usually their fears are unwarranted, and with a reassuring explanation they will proceed with the roentgenograms.

X-rays should always include the standard views plus special views as indicated for a particular injury. Occasionally comparison of x-rays of the opposite side is necessary to confirm an undisplaced fracture, or confirm a growth pattern, or observe some anomaly in the patient. If arthritis is manifested in one extremity and is alleged to be due to the injury, x-rays should be taken of the opposite side to learn if there is similar arthritis in the uninjured extremity.

X-rays should be taken periodically to demonstrate any progression of a pre-existing condition such as arthritis as a result of the accident. If there are x-ray changes visible at the time of the initial injury, it is presumed that they antedated the injury. Follow-up x-rays six or twelve months later which show little change, would indicate no permanent traumatic aggravation of the pre-existing condition. On the other hand, if there is a considerable increase in sclerosis, spurring, narrowing of the joint space, cystic formation, etc., more than one would anticipate with the passage of time, then the examiner can state that the arthritis has been aggravated by the accident (Figure 9).

Physicians who frequently examine laborers or workmen involved in strenuous occupations, have noted a rather high incidence of hypertrophic spurring in the lumbar spine. Those engaged in occupations requiring constant kneeling and working in that position, for example, carpet layers or tile artisans, demonstrate a high incidence of calcification of the quadriceps tendon insertion and spurring in the knees, particularly of the inferior margins of the patella. This represents a response to repeated injury, with calcareous deposits in the repeatedly traumatized quadriceps or patellar tendon, also the margins of the patella. Similar spurs are occasionally noted in the tibial spines for the same reasons. The presence of such spurring does not necessarily indicate osteoarthritis, but rather a physiological response to occupational trauma. Usually these findings are

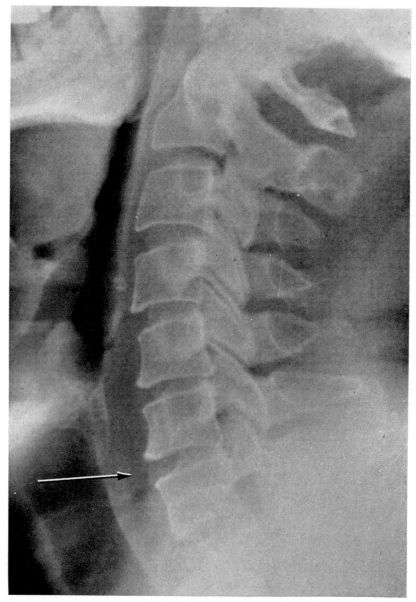

FIGURE 9. TRAUMATIC AGGRAVATION OF PRE-EXISTING
ARTHRITIS.
A. 1. Cervical spine, 10-21-66 (day of injury). Minute speck of calci-
fication in the anterior longitudinal ligament at C-6-7.

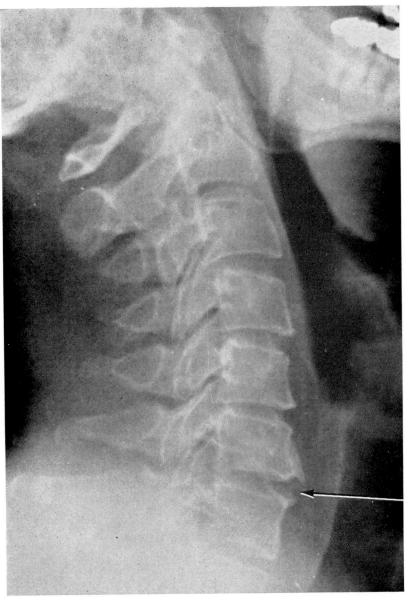

A. 2. X-rays, 10-19-67 (one year after accident). Considerable calcification in the anterior spinal ligament with spurs C-6-7. The degree of calcification and degenerative change exceeds that anticipated after the passage of one year's time. Definite evidence of traumatic aggravation demonstrated on these films. Normal lordotic curve present.

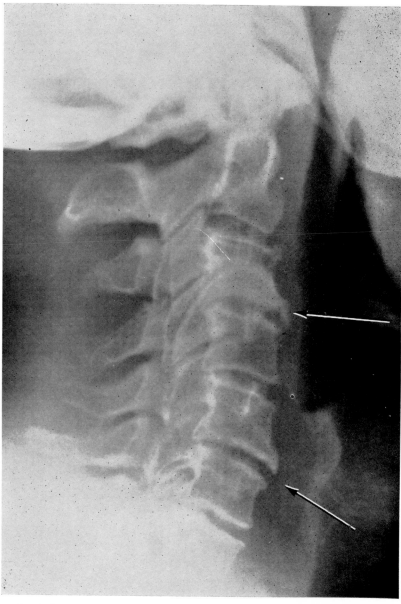

B. 1. X-rays, 7-20-66 (day of injury). Spurring noted at C-3, 4, 5, and 6, with minimal narrowing of interspaces C-3-4 and C-5-6. Note reversal of lordotic curve in upper half of cervical spine with neck extended.

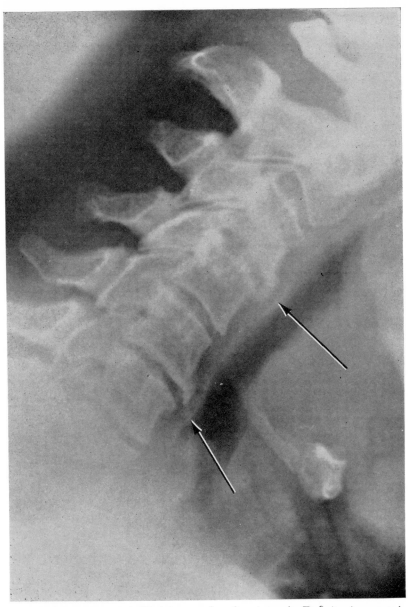

B. 2. X-rays, 1-3-67 (six months after injury). Definite increase in narrowing and sclerosis at C-3-4, with marked increase in spurring here; slight increase in spurring at C-5-6, with increased narrowing of the interspace. Changes are significant as they appeared within five months of injury, demonstrating rapid acceleration of degenerative changes, in excess of that anticipated within said period of time. Lordotic curve obliterated with neck flexed forward, indicating absence of muscle spasm.

asymptomatic and are detected by x-ray examination performed for a superimposed injury.

Although it is preferable for the examining physician to review personally all x-rays, this procedure is not always practical, especially if the x-rays have been taken in other cities; in cases like these a report may be secured by telephone or by letter. However, if the x-rays have been interpreted by a Board-certified roentgenologist at a hospital or in private practice, the report may be quoted, especially if it is negative. Whenever degenerative changes such as arthritis are reported and there is a question of traumatic aggravation, it is good policy to secure the initial x-rays for personal evaluation and comparison with later films taken by the examiner, before findings are quoted, as there is considerable variation in diagnostic terms and the interpretation of degenerative arthritis.

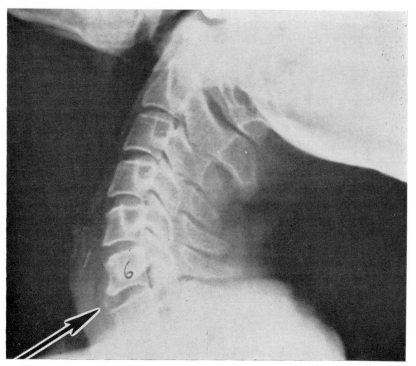

C. 1. X-rays, 6-19-67 (nine months after injury). Minimal calcification of the anterior spinal ligament, C-6-7.

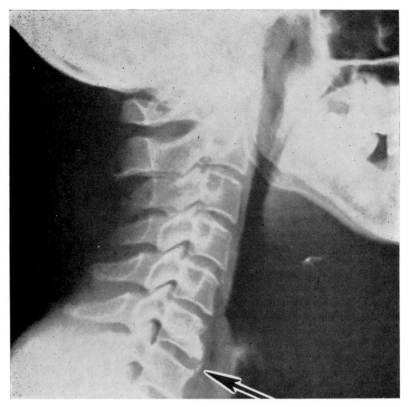

C. 2. X-ray, 10-19-67 (fifteen months after injury). Definite spurring and increased calcification at C-6-7, indicating accelerated degenerative changes.

If the initial x-rays showed some straightening of the lordotic curve in the cervical and lumbar areas, and subsequent x-rays made by the examiner showed a normal curve, this may or may not confirm the presence of muscle spasm shortly after the accident, but it would demonstrate that the apparent muscle spasm is no longer present, as the normal curve had been restored to the spine. On the witness stand the doctor may be questioned regarding soft tissue injuries which were not revealed by x-ray. He should be prepared to testify that most soft tissue injuries are not apparent by x-ray and that a negative x-ray examination does not signify absence of injury.

Occasionally a joint effusion, such as in the knee, can be demonstrated by soft tissue x-ray technique. Tears of the collateral ligaments can be demonstrated as widening of the joint space with special stress films; these are films taken with the knee relaxed, and then with the knee strongly abducted and adducted.

Reports of Previous X-rays

Reports of x-rays taken by a general practitioner in his own office are of limited value and cannot be given the same weight as reports from an approved x-ray laboratory, although many general practitioners are adept in x-ray interpretation.

Information concerning previous x-rays may often be secured over the telephone but, if at all lengthy, should be followed by a written report. This procedure facilitates the immediate examination and determines the need for additional x-rays, which can then be taken without delay. It may be necessary to have the patient sign a routine consent form to obtain the previous x-rays, especially if the x-rays were taken at a government agency such as a Veterans Administration or military installation, where regulations prohibit forwarding of information without the written consent of the patient.

Loss of Lordotic Curve by X-ray

Reports of x-ray studies of the cervical and lumbar spine may sometimes include a statement that "there has been a loss of the normal lordotic curve which indicates the presence of muscle spasm." This interpretation has been made by radiologists, orthopaedists, and other physicians treating patients with neck and low back injuries (See Figure 9). Because of the increased credence given x-ray reports as objective evidence, such an interpretation lends considerable support to the plaintiff's case by indicating an unquestionably severe injury. The plaintiff's attorney will undoubtedly use this statement in the presentation of his case in court, especially in the cross-examination of a defendant witness who has stated he could find no evidence of injury at the time of his examination. He will also try to elicit from that witness a statement that there must have been a severe initial injury in order to cause the loss of the normal lordotic curve; favorable evidence from an opposing witness will greatly strengthen his case.

However, it has been well documented that straightening of the spine particularly in the cervical region, does not necessarily indicate there is a loss of the normal lordotic curve due to muscle spasm resulting from a severe soft tissue injury. Most experienced examiners who have noted the presence of a straight cervical curve on x-rays taken after a completely negative clinical examination, have discounted the x-ray findings because of the lack of any supporting clinical evidence.

Numerous scientific papers have reported on the clinical significance of a straight cervical spine as seen on lateral x-rays taken in the neutral position. Johl, Muller and Roberts found a straight or reverse pattern of the cervical spine on the lateral roentgenograms of 46 out of 116 normal patients; they found an even higher frequency of straightening when the subject held himself in the position of "military attention," i.e. retraction of the chin without flexion of the neck, and with voluntary contracture of the neck musculature. Threadgill also noted that it was possible for a patient to straighten his neck during the examination and produce straightening of the cervical spine on lateral roentgenogram.[35]

Fineman and his group[9] reviewed lateral roentgenograms of the cervical spine of 330 patients varying from age 17 to age 77, at Montefiore and Flower-Fifth Avenue Hospital, New York City. X-rays were made with the neck in the neutral position, but sixty-one, or 19 per cent, showed a straight cervical spine; twelve of the sixty-one patients had a history of injury to the neck; forty-nine had no history of any trauma which would have accounted for the loss of lordotic curve. These researchers noted considerable variations in the posture of patients from positioning by the x-ray technician; they also observed variation in the heights of the chin and inclination of the cervical spine which would cause some straightening.

Fineman's group compared 129 routine lateral roentgenograms

with 129 made with the chin lowered. Fifty-three, or 41 per cent of the patients, showed a loss of cervical lordosis, straightening of the curve or reversal of the curve. Fifty-three showed no loss of the lordotic curve and twenty-three showed a linear or kyphotic pattern. Of the fifty-three patients with a change of curve, forty, or 75 per cent, gave no history of injury to the neck, and only thirteen, or 25 per cent, gave a history of recent injury.

The following conclusions were reached:
1. A straightened cervical spine or even a slight kyphosis may be associated with cervical spondylosis deformans.
2. A straightened or kyphotic cervical spine may occur normally.
3. A change from a lordotic to a linear pattern or to a kyphotic pattern may result from slight variation in the positioning of the patient for the lateral roentgenograms, such as the lowered chin position.
4. A straightened or kyphotic cervical spine as seen on lateral roentgenograms, does not necessarily indicate muscle spasm due to injury of the cervical spine.

This study supports the clinical observations of many orthopaedists that the loss or reversal of a lordotic curve does not necessarily reflect a recent injury. The positioning of the patient, the use of varying techniques of different x-ray technicians, the normal variations in the appearance of the cervical spine, or the presence of pre-existing degenerative arthritic changes—all may cause a loss of the normal lordotic curve without any type of injury. The report of a change or reversal of the curve in 75 per cent of the cases studied, in which there was no history of any injury whatsoever to the neck, is certainly significant. The expert medical witness may use this data in his interpretation of lateral cervical spine x-rays to support his opinions when questioned on the witness stand.[31]

X-rays in Children

X-ray plates of the cervical spine in children must be properly interpreted before diagnosing an injury following an accident, especially one in which there is a history of injury to the neck with resultant pain and stiffness. It has been well established that x-rays may show a variation in the epiphyses and vertebral anatomy, incomplete ossification of cartilaginous centers, and hypermobility of the cervical spine. Subluxation, the displacement of one vertebra on another, particularly in the upper cervical spine, and the loss of lordosis of the cervical spine in the neutral position, may be the result of injuries causing spasm of the para-vertebral muscles, but this interpretation is not unequivocally true. Unlike the situation in cases of injuries to the extremities, there is here no contralateral extremity available for a comparison x-ray to aid in the diagnosis.

Cattell and Filtzer[5] made a study of 160 children to determine normal variations in the cervical spine to aid in diagnosis. They noted atlanto-axial mobility, variations of the cervical spine curve in flexion, congenital abnormalities, and epiphyseal variations as previously reported. An apparent subluxation between the bodies of C-2,3, observed when the spine was flexed but not seen in extension, was graphically demonstrated in their article, but they concluded that this was actually a pseudo-subluxation and not the result of injury. They further concluded that the variations were manifestations of an immature skeleton, hypermobility, unique vertebral configuration or incomplete ossification, and single or multiple epiphyses, all of which contribute to the difficulty in interpreting roentgenograms of the cervical spine in children. Experienced observers have noted that the symptoms will rapidly disappear when it is not the result of trauma, even though the variation persists, indicating that the variation is a normal one for that individual. This was also noted by Cattell and Filtzer.

In a patient with a mild x-ray abnormality, the necessity for treatment would be indicated by continued muscle spasm, limited motion, or a torticollis, deformed position of the head and neck, and *not* by the x-ray finding alone. Overtreatment of a child may result in a psychological impact, and can be avoided in favor of a more conservative approach, if normal variations are recognized and x-rays properly interpreted. It is important that physicians who care for children with neck injuries be familiar with the normal roentgenographic variations.

Hypertrophic Changes—Osteoarthritis

Mild hypertrophic changes, such as minimal spurs, are frequently found in patients over forty years of age, particularly in the spine or extremities of individuals who have been engaged in arduous labor over long periods of time. Spurring, sclerosis, and small degrees of calcification in the anterior spinal ligaments, of either the cervical or lumbar areas, may be observed in hard-working laborers, and construction men in their late 30's or 40's; usually such changes are not seen until the late 50's or in older age groups. Similarly, as we have already noted, changes may be observed in the knees of individuals doing a considerable amount of kneeling, among them carpet and floor layers, cement masons, etc. The constant stress of their occupation places a strain upon the bones and associated ligaments and joints, and produces the wear-and-tear phenomena commonly associated with degenerative changes. However, this observation does not necessarily signify an arthritic change, but merely common physiological changes which are accelerated by the strain of a particular trade or occupation.

It is generally considered incorrect to diagnose such changes as a true clinical entity of osteoarthritis. Several authors have used the term *osteophytosis* in order to differentiate between physiological osteophytes or spurs, and true arthritis. In most instances these changes are present without symptoms and are not responsible for the patient's complaints. The inexperienced physician may ascribe a patient's extreme discomfort and disability to such changes when the real reason may be functional in nature. Such an error will lead to unnecessary and improper treatment, which may increase the patient's functional symptoms and maximize his feelings of disability. Accurate diagnosis is needed to avoid needless disputes in a case which might otherwise be promptly settled.

The procurement of x-ray reports is not always a simple matter. Many hospitals are conscious of their medico-legal nature and refuse to give any information without written authorization. These regulations may not only delay treatment, but also lead to repetitious x-rays, which would be unnecessary if the report of the initial x-rays had been promptly secured. The doctor cannot proceed with treatment without a full knowledge of the extent of injury, and yet he is thwarted in securing information. This is particularly true in hospitals operated by federal, state or municipal authorities, which frequently have strict regulations forbidding release of information without proper authorization.

The failure to secure a full report of the x-rays in the case may lead to overlooking proper diagnoses and to delay in administering correct and needed treatment. An example of one such incident follows: A child was brought to the office after an automobile accident with multiple but apparently minor injuries. The parents, who were not too well informed, had no knowledge of the extent of the patient's injuries and had been given little information. After examination at the hospital, the child was sent home. The initial request for x-ray information from the hospital x-ray laboratory had been denied, with the statement that the reports would be sent upon receipt of written authorization. However, the attending physician (a member of the hospital staff), suspicious of injuries which had not been treated, contacted the Chief of Service, who later called and informed him that the child had suffered a fracture of the clavicle that had not been treated, but had been discovered after the child's release. The doctor then recalled the patient to his office and instituted proper treatment.

In this instance both the hospital and the doctor could have been subjected to a malpractice claim had proper treatment not been promptly instituted. Thus, though there are medico-legal implications for release of medical information, sometimes there are overriding considerations which necessitate prompt release of information to responsible individuals.

Value of X-rays in Defendant Examinations

In recent years there has been increased awareness of x-ray radiation, resulting in occasional objections to the taking of x-rays.

Although unnecessary exposure should be avoided, it is the claimant who has initiated the litigation, and the defendant is entitled to all possible evidence in defense of that claim. Occasionally, the claimant will refuse to have x-rays taken by the defendant examiner, stating that he has already had too many x-rays taken, which may be true. However, the examiner fully realizes that it may be difficult or impossible to obtain the x-rays taken by the plaintiff's physician, because of the lack of cooperation from that person's attorney or physician. Such a patient is frequently associated with an unjustified claim, grossly exaggerates injuries, and makes excessive demands for compensation. The individual who has a just claim, on the other hand, is usually cooperative and understanding, and the case is disposed of without prolonged litigation.

The defendant examiner has only one opportunity to take the x-rays, as generally only one defendant examination is permitted, and even this sometimes requires a court order. It is rare that an opportunity for a second examination is given to the defendant physician. If circumstances warrant, it should be explained to the patient (female in this instance) that the dangers of excessive radiation are minimal and that a protective apron will be used over her abdomen while x-rays are being taken of her neck and extremities. If she still refuses x-ray examination, she should be advised to call her attorney or treating physician for permission to have the x-rays *before* leaving the office, if at all possible, as a promise to return later is rarely kept.

It is important that x-rays be made even though it is anticipated that they will be negative, as this documentation will strengthen the doctor's evidence when he responds to questions on cross-examination. The court and jury place considerable weight on x-ray findings, which are considered strong objective evidence. If no x-rays have been made in the prior six months and the patient has continuing complaints, the doctor should insist upon further x-rays in order to corroborate his opinion, especially if his clinical examination has been entirely negative.

In a recent case, a youth with multiple fractures had been extensively x-rayed two days previously by his treating physician, who was preparing a final evaluation and report. The defendant examiner informed the mother that he would prefer to obtain the other doctor's x-rays rather than repeat them, which is good clinical judgment. A telephone call was made to the treating physician, and he agreed to release the films to the mother, who promised to bring them to the examiner's office the following morning for personal review and immediate return to her physician. The mother never appeared at the office the following day, and the doctor did not see the x-rays because she had, in the meantime, called her attorney who forbade release of the films.

This incident illustrates how important it is for the examiner to have his own x-rays; he needs them not only to complete his report but also to have on hand for presentation at trial if necessary. The additional radiation exposure is a responsibility of the claimant and one of the liabilities that he must incur when he pursues a litigation claim. If the patient refuses x-ray examination, this refusal can be put in evidence and will not be favorable to the plaintiff's case.

Myelograms

The myelogram is a valuable adjunct for diagnosis of the etiology of pain in the low back and neck. It is now an established procedure in the diagnosis of a herniated disc syndrome in the cervical and lumbar areas. Laminectomy is rarely performed without a preliminary myelographic study; this determines not only the presence of a disc but also its specific location, and thus facilitates surgery.

It is generally recognized that the myelogram is not 100 per cent accurate and is positive in only 80 to 85 per cent of cases where there is a definite herniation of the disc. In other words, 15 to 20 per cent of individuals who are suffering from definite disc protrusion and who require surgery, will not demonstrate a defect on a myelogram. Thus the diagnosis must be based on the patient's history and an objective examination as well as on myelographic evidence. In cases where the clinical evidence is positive, the physician should rely on his clinical judgment and proceed with treatment despite a negative myelogram.

In some instances, the myelogram may give a false positive result—i.e. there is a defect with no actual clinical disease or injury present. Again the results must be evaluated and compared to the clinical examination and history. Spinal fluid is withdrawn at the time of the myelogram and can be sent for complete laboratory analysis, including the protein content (which is increased in tumors), a colloidal gold curve (which is indicative of degenerative changes of the spinal cord such as multiple sclerosis), tests for syphilis, cell count (which may indicate infection), and glucose and chloride analysis.

Hitzelberger and Witten, writing in the *Journal of Neurosurgery* of Chicago in March 1969, reviewed 300 patients who had myelograms performed primarily for detection of cranial lesions involving the posterior fossa; none of these patients had any symptoms referable to the neck or lower back. However, in 37 per cent of the examinations, the findings reflected an abnormality in the disc; 19 per cent showed a single abnormality and 24 per cent a multiple abnormality; most of the defects were in the lumbar region. Twenty-one per cent had an abnormality of the cervical spine and 8 per cent had defects in both the lumbar and cervical areas. This study emphasizes that false positive results do occur in significant percentages which must be recognized in evaluating a positive myelogram.

It is not generally recognized by most surgeons that frequent false positive findings are associated with a myelographic study. Hour-glass types of constrictions, in the absence of supporting clinical findings, and a defect about the area of the needle insertion (usually an artifact) are generally recognized as not representing a significant clinical abnormality; this study indicates an even higher incidence of defects demonstrated by the myelogram which are not due to actual clinical pathology. The study emphasizes that the myelogram is only an adjunct in diagnosis which is not infallible in the evaluation of a nerve compression syndrome in either the lumbar or cervical regions.

DEFENDANT'S EXAMINATIONS

Defendant examinations sometimes present special problems although the great majority are performed in a routine fashion and without incident. The majority of claimants are honest and cooperative and can be examined without false claims of injury or restrictions related to their examination. Problems arise usually with the claimant who is exaggerating and has continued to complain despite extensive and proper treatment by his or her own physician. More than the usual allotted time is required for such an examination.

Obnoxious Patients

The doctor may be irritated by bizarre behavior in uncooperative patients, such as pushing his hand away when he attempts to palpate the area of alleged tenderness, or warning the doctor, "Don't you hurt me, don't bend my back, don't twist my neck," and so on. These individuals are hostile, obviously on the defensive, with a *chip on the shoulder* attitude; they are probably reporting for an examination only because they are required to do so. Many are either neurotic or consciously promoting a claim for monetary gain. Should the doctor lose his patience and state he will not tolerate the patient's objectionable behavior, the patient may dress and leave the office without permitting further examination. This will be to no one's advantage, and the situation should be avoided. The doctor must remember that you cannot treat an abnormal person in a normal fashion; this truth is just as applicable in coping with these individuals as in dealing with known psychotic patients. The doctor should be tolerant and patient, complete the examination, and get the objectionable patient out of the office as quickly as possible. Some of the hostility in these claimants may have been engendered by the patient's attorney who often instructs the patient to be negativistic and uncooperative.

An extreme example is provided in the following incident in which an orthopaedist was asked to examine a female patient who had recently undergone anterior cervical spine fusion. The doctor was provided with an inch-thick file of medical reports and hospital records which he reviewed prior to the examination date. When the patient appeared for the examination, she handed him a written statement outlining her history and also a copy of a court order which limited his examination. The doctor had never been faced with such instructions and his first reaction was to cancel the examination and withdraw from the case. However, realizing that this unorthodox beginning was a challenge and that perhaps he could be of considerable help to the defendant attorney, he decided to proceed with the examination. He knew the defendant attorney well, having performed multiple surgery upon his son to correct deformities of poliomyelitis, and he did not want to "let him down."

Here is the letter which was signed by both the patient and her husband. The accompanying legal document follows.

April 26, 1971

Dear Dr. Ames,

While we have consented to this examination by you on behalf of the Defendant, and will cooperate in every way, we have been concerned about any physical examination so soon following the surgery. Therefore, our attorney secured an order of court concerning the examination. Your attention is specifically invited to this order of court, a certified copy of which is attached to this letter.

Our attorney has requested that we submit a written history to you in order that there be no confusion about the facts. He has also requested that we answer any questions you may ask.

On December 9, 1969, I was stopped at the corner of Wisconsin and Massachusetts Ave., in Washington, D.C., when my car stalled. When I attempted to start it, I was struck from behind by another automobile. I was driving an Opel Kadet Station Wagon and the striking car was a Cadillac sedan. The rear of my car was damaged. I secured two estimates for the repair, the lowest of which was $250.00. At impact I did not lose consciousness, but I did notice immediate pain in my neck, with no radiation into my shoulders. The pain became quite severe that evening, and I had difficulty sleeping. On December 10, 1969, the pain continued. I was not otherwise hurt.

At age fifteen or sixteen, I was a passenger in an automobile accident and was hospitalized with facial injuries. Later my nose was the subject of surgery. I also had pain in my lower back for about two years, but was not troubled with back pain after that. I have never had any difficulty with my neck before the accident of December 9, 1969.

I saw Dr. Francis Day on December 11, 1969, and have continued under his care since that time. He has prescribed various medications, traction, a supporting collar, and physical therapy. I tried to work at my job as a school teacher following the accident, having returned to work on January 15, 1970 or thereabouts. However, the discomfort was so great that Dr. Day stopped my working toward the end of that month, and I have been unable to work since that time.

While trying to teach during January 1970, I developed burning pain in both of my shoulders. My neck was stiff and it hurt to move it. This grew worse and I developed a stinging pain in my upper back and some pain down the back of my left leg. I could hardly move my left shoulder because of pain. As a result of these problems, Dr. Day hospitalized me at Sibley Hospital on February 1, 1970, where I remained until February 9, 1970. While there, traction and physiotherapy were applied.

Upon my return home I developed numbness in both upper arms and pain around the shoulder blades in addition to my other symptoms. Dr. Day performed certain examinations. The results of these are contained in his reports which have been furnished to the attorney who has employed you in this case. My symptoms during the year of 1970 would get better then worse—anytime I participated in any significant household activities, for example, the symptoms would become much worse. Dr. Day had me admitted to Georgetown Hospital for a myelogram on December 5, 1970, and I was discharged on December 10th. Thereafter I was given electromyogram tests at Dr. Day's directions. On February 20, 1971, Dr. Day performed an anterior cervical fusion at the Georgetown University Hospital.

My symptoms have been improved since that surgery in that the constant pain previously present is now absent. Needless to say I look forward to resuming a more normal life with my family as soon as possible, consistent with my recovery from my injuries, and resultant surgery. But it has only been a few weeks since I left the hospital.

Very truly yours,
Angela Devon
Leon Devon

IN THE CIRCUIT COURT FOR PRINCE GEORGE'S COUNTY
STATE OF MARYLAND
Sitting as a Court of Law

ANGELA DEVON, et al)
     Plaintiffs   )
vs.   )   Law No. 58.926
JACK HOUSTON   )
     Defendant   )

ORDER

Upon consideration of Defendant's Motion for Medical Examination of Plaintiff and Plaintiff's Response thereto, and after hearing, it is, this 31st day of March, 1971, by the Circuit Court of Prince George's County, State of Maryland, Sitting as a Court of Law,

ORDERED, That the Plaintiff, Angela Devon, submit to a medical examination by Dr. Joseph Ames, M.D., at a time mutually convenient to the parties, and it is further

ORDERED, That the said physical examination shall not include any twisting, moving, or bending of the Plaintiff's neck and cervical spine, and it is further

ORDERED, That the Defense shall provide Plaintiff's counsel with a written report of the examining doctor's findings and conclusions at least five (5) days before the date of trial.

Lucas Daniels
Judge of the Circuit Court for
Prince George's County, State of Maryland

During the examination, which was witnessed by the husband, the doctor exercised extreme caution, as her fear of injury from a strenuous examination was realistic, inasmuch as she had been operated upon only five weeks previously. The examination should have been postponed to a later date, but her trial was to be held in two weeks. In accordance with the order that he was not to twist, move, or bend the plaintiff's neck and cervical spine, he did not measure the range of motion with the Cervigon apparatus, but instead had the patient remove her cervical collar, and then asked her to move her head and neck without touching her, and with no passive assistance from the examiner. He then estimated the active motion but did not make any accurate measurements.

At trial, the plaintiff's attorney sharply criticized the doctor for having disobeyed the court order by examining her neck, although he had merely observed her moving it, which she had done at his request but voluntarily. The doctor noted that she could have refused to do so. The plaintiff attorney, noted for the sharpness of his cross examination and for his hostility toward expert defendant witnesses, insisted that the doctor had violated a court order because of this procedure. It was the physician's understanding that the patient should be able to perform any motions of which she was capable as long as he did not force her into any maneuver. This of course was an extreme example of hostility and an attempt to intimidate an expert medical witness.

In this particular case, the treating physician had been hospitalized for mental problems a short time after performing the anterior cervical fusion. The operation had been performed despite a negative consultation by a competent neurosurgeon who refused to perform any surgery in this case because of a negative myelogram, x-rays, and other tests. The defendant orthopaedist testified that he did not believe the patient had required surgery. When asked on cross examination whether he believed the operation should not have been performed, he answered in the affirmative, and reiterated the basis of his opinion, including the previously mentioned negative findings. This was a difficult position for the witness, but it was clearly evident the operation should not have been performed. Incidentally, the neurosurgeon who had refused to operate, one of the most prominent in the community, was never called as a witness by the plaintiff.

After the witness left the stand, an attorney conference was held and the case was settled for a substantially lower figure than the plaintiff's demand. The settlement figure, however, was still quite high, as the patient had incurred great expenses and had undergone major surgery which required a prolonged recovery period. This was a direct result of the accident, as she would not have undergone surgery had she not been involved in the accident; the fact that the surgery was not indicated was a matter between the patient and her surgeon, and did not exclude the defendant from the responsibility for that surgery, if his liability was established.

This case demonstrates that the doctor who performs frequent defendant examinations must be prepared on occasion to encounter unusual situations and to meet arduous demands upon his patience and understanding. When faced with a court order, he must comply and follow its instructions or otherwise be subjected to a cause of action. Although the situation may be irritating, he should complete the examination without delay and not concern himself with the intricacies of litigation.

Harassment of Defendant Examiner

The physician who performs defendant examinations may be subjected to harassment from the patient's attorney if his report is unfavorable to his client. The examiner should write an objective report clearly stating his findings and opinions. Ordinarily this is accepted by the plaintiff's attorney, who will respect his opinion, even though it may be unfavorable and at variance with the reports of his treating physician. However, an inexperienced plaintiff's attorney, particularly one who practices negligence law only occasionally, may resent a strong negative report and forward letters to the insurance company or the doctor attacking his integrity and competence. In contrast, attorneys who have a large negligence practice are frequently familiar with the established reputation of the defendant's physician and do not object to a statement of his true opinion.

A physician who examines and treats a large number of plaintiffs but also performs frequent defendant examinations may be respected by referring attorneys as an honest and fair examiner.

who does not take a stand on "either side of the fence." However, any physician who performs a great number of defendant examinations will be subjected to some harassment sooner or later, resulting from the frequent incidence of neuroses and exaggeration in plaintiffs, which culminates in complaints to their attorneys for strong action against "that nasty, hostile physician." The doctor may receive a letter attacking his integrity or making vicious statements about his ability, often claiming that "he only spent two minutes with me," "he hardly touched me as he was busy on the telephone all the time he was in the room," and so forth. Of course, the attorney was not present during the examination and has only the self-serving word of his client. However, in some instances, he may threaten a lawsuit for malpractice or alleged injuries sustained by his client as the result of the "strenuous examination." An example of such reactions is noted in the following communications.

Dear Dr. Brown:

With reference to your perfunctory examination of my client, Joan Doe, on December 11, 1960, please be advised that the undersigned considers your attitude and behavior deplorable.

Certainly, it must have occurred to you—from past experiences—that not all patients examined by your office for the benefit of liability carriers have been "whiplash willies" trying to make a buck. Your ostensible findings that Miss Doe's neck will rotate fully, and the back will bend properly regardless of pain—is quite an empirical revelation.

I consider your approach to matters of this nature as teetering on professional malpractice and therefore am considering what further action, if any, is required.

Sincerely,
John Black, Esq.

Dear Dr. Brown:

I have been retained by Mrs. Mildred Crow for the purpose of recovering from you damages sustained by her on February 1, 1966, when Mrs. Crow sustained injuries in the course of an examination conducted by you.

If you are insured, I recommend that you immediately refer this matter to your insurance carrier. If you are not insured, and desire to discuss this matter further, I recommend that you call me at your earliest convenience. Should I not hear from either you or your insurance company within a reasonable period of time, I shall, on behalf of Mrs. Crow, institute legal proceedings against you.

> Very truly yours,
> Milton Taupe, Esq.

Such letters would most likely be prejudicial to the plaintiff's case, if admitted in evidence at trial, but defendant attorneys do not want to add any additional problems to their case and usually advise the examiner to *forget it.* Fortunately, these incidents occur infrequently and are not condoned by reputable members of the legal profession.

One of the hazards of defense examinations is the attitude of a hostile patient who reports for examination against his wish. Such a patient, as well as the neurotic patient, often refuses to give any information regarding his accident or medical care and makes it obvious he resents the whole examination procedure. This will be apparent to the examining physician after he begins his history-taking. After the examination, or sometimes during the examination, such a patient will allege that a doctor has hurt him as a result of examination procedures, despite the utmost caution and care exercised by the physician. It is good practice to have an assistant present as a witness when this type of patient is encountered, in order to defend against any possible later allegations of injury or maltreatment. In addition, the doctor should be very cautious in dictating his findings in the hearing of such a patient; it is preferable to make notes and dictate later, or else leave the room and dictate out of the presence of the patient.

If the doctor suspects that a claim for maltreatment will be made, as ascertained from the patient's attitude and remarks during the examination, he should mention this in his report, noting that the patient may allege that he was injured by his examination. He should emphasize the caution and care exercised during the examination and give his opinion whether any actual injury was sustained. Further evidence may be obtained by performing some of the tests for malingering, to note if there is any anatomical association of complaints with the examining maneuvers.

Not infrequently, the patient will continue to complain bitterly after a maneuver like toe flexion and extension in the prone position, claiming such severe back pain that he can hardly get dressed and leave the office. Of course the patient does not realize that the muscles that flex and extend the toes originate below the knee, and could not possibly have any influence on his low back musculature, ligaments, or joints! The following letters regarding Helen Bloe offer an excellent example of such a situation.

Mr. Joseph Money
Claim Department
Willoughby Casualty and Surety Co.
Rockville, Maryland

Dear Mr. Money:
Thank you for your recent letter of January 28, 1965, and returned herewith is the check for $600.00. We appreciate your good intention but my client does not wish to accept it.
I was quite appalled to learn that when Mrs. Bloe went to be examined by the doctor which the insurance company chose, the doctor allegedly had her do sit ups which caused her pain, thereby causing her to have to return to her own doctor for treatment. Mrs. Bloe's doctor has stated that this aggravated her injury and he has had to put her in traction.

With kind regards,
John Crenshaw, Esq.

Certified #1043

Dear Dr. Brown:
Please be advised that the undersigned is the attorney for Mrs. Helen Bloe. Would you please give me the name of your insurance carrier who represents you on your malpractice suits. Mrs. Bloe intends to bring action against you and she alleges that due to the fact that you gave her strenuous exercises to do when you examined her, you aggravated her injuries and she was recently readmitted to Brownsville Hospital. Thank you in advance for this consideration.

Sincerely,
John Crenshaw, Esq.

In this instance, the patient returned to her treating physician with a report of the doctor's "vicious examination and assault" which caused her an enormous amount of low back discomfort. Her physician immediately placed her in a local hospital (incidentally, he was a principal stockholder in that private hospital) and administered further treatment over a period of several weeks. By coincidence the defendant doctor had some advance information regarding this situation from a former patient who was employed at the hospital and to whom the plaintiff had related her problems.

In cases of this type there is often a strong element of anxiety with a long history of unresponsive, multi-phasic and continued complaints for many months or years. The treating physician should be well aware of this problem from his close contact with the patient, and should evaluate the latter's complaints following a defense examination in accordance with his or her neurotic tendencies. However, not all physicians are considerate of their confreres, and some have no compunction in increasing their medical bill by administering treatment as desired by the patient, whether or not it is indicated. On the other hand, the treating physician is burdened with a difficult patient with many complaints and he may administer some treatment, even though he suspects there is no factual basis for the complaints, in order to relieve an unpleasant situation. However, if the treating physician takes a firm stand, which is frequently done by reputable doctors, and informs the patient that there is no real basis for his complaints and he does not require any further treatment, the case can often be quickly settled, and the doctor is relieved of his problem. Letters with the threat of possible malpractice action may represent an attempt to coerce the doctor for more favorable reports in future examinations or to soften the impact of his testimony in that particular case. Obviously these tactics should not have any influence on the doctor's opinion, reports, or testimony.

After the above incident, the defendant physician felt compelled to notify his malpractice insurance carrier. He wrote the following letter:

I am enclosing a copy of a recent letter which is self-explanatory. I mentioned something about this case to you when you were in my office recently. At this point I do not intend to answer this letter unless you advise me otherwise.

The reference is to a sitting-up maneuver which was performed in the examination performed for the defendant, Sentinel Insurance Company. The examination was conducted without removing a back brace which the patient wore to my office; she advised me that her surgeon had instructed her not to remove the support at any time. The patient stated that she was unable to bend forward in the standing position more than 10 to 15 degrees. She was then asked to sit on the examining table, which she did with her knees fully extended. She was then asked to bend forward to try to touch her toes, to go as far as possible. This was done by the patient without any help from me, without me touching the patient. She did it one time only, not repeatedly. She was able to bend forward flexing her back to a right angle, thereby demonstrating that she did have much more motion than she cared to demonstrate in the erect position. The patient did not make any mention of having pain when doing this, stating only that this was as far as she could bend (which was far enough to demonstrate my point). It should be noted that this is a definite orthopaedic examining maneuver and she was not asked to perform any sitting-up exercises as alleged by Mr. Crenshaw in a previous letter to the Sentinel Insurance Company. I enclose a copy of an examining form devised by Dr. Earl McBride of Oklahoma, which has been widely distributed throughout the orthopaedic world; Dr. McBride is well known for his work on disability evaluation. You are referred to Figure X, which is the maneuver involved. I believe this is self-explanatory. I cannot conceive of any manner in which there could be any negligence or malpractice. Obviously the problem arose when my negative examination report was received by the plaintiff's attorney. Please advise me if you wish me to furnish any further information.

After the letter was sent, the doctor was contacted by his malpractice carrier and this did influence his coverage, as he had another claim outstanding because of the alleged negligence of a previous associate. The threat of another claim adversely affected the attitude of his carrier, but unfortunately his insurance coverage was continued. There was further action in the case after the negligence case was settled.

The above incident illustrates a significant hazard in performing defense examinations, as adverse letters to the doctor's malpractice carrier jeopardize his coverage and may increase his rates, even though the threatening actions are unwarranted. Even the threat of a malpractice action impairs the image of the physician, despite the lack of a true basis for the complaint, as once the allegation and complaint is made, the doctor always suffers some damage, either to his reputation or to his "nervous system." In addition it necessitates correspondence and time which could otherwise be devoted to his medical practice.

The defendant's doctor may also be annoyed by anonymous phone calls to his office or home from unhappy plaintiffs he has recently examined. His receptionist may be bombarded with repeated blank calls which she must routinely answer, often to the detriment of normal office routine. This usually occurs for several days after the hostile or neurotic plaintiff leaves the office with the knowledge that the examiner had not been impressed with his various complaints.

In recent years the malpractice problem has become a very serious one and defense examinations increase the already extensive hazards of medical practice. As a result fewer physicians of established reputation will accept referrals from insurance companies for defendant evaluations, despite the assured payment of satisfactory fees for their professional services. The examinations require a considerable amount of the doctor's limited appointment time, and a significant number of these appointments are not kept. Most busy specialists do not want the annoyances of trial alerts, lost appointment time, last minute cancellation of testimony, review of extensive records, and undesirable hostile plaintiffs; the monetary gain rarely compensates the doctor for the many inconveniences and increased stress placed on his private practice.

Harassment of an expert witness may involve any personal or professional incident in his life which the opposing attorney believes will have a derogatory effect on the witness' character or reputation. If the witness has a court record of civil or criminal offenses, or domestic problems, an attempt may be made to insert these factors into the trial proceedings; however, usually an objection is made and sustained by the court.

Because medical malpractice has affected many physicians, an occasional attorney has used a previous malpractice action as a vehicle to embarrass a medical expert on the witness stand. A malpractice suit becomes part of the public record and any attorney can learn the facts by consulting court files. He can then use the circumstances and results of this legal action to tarnish the reputation of the witness. However, the court may uphold an objection to such evidence as being irrelevant.

Such an incident did occur in Georgia, in the course of which the court refused to permit further questions of an expert medical witness regarding a previous malpractice action.

While taking an oral deposition the physician was asked questions regarding his qualifications as well as the treatment and diagnosis of the patient under his care. He was questioned about a previous malpractice suit; he answered several questions and acknowledged that a judgment was secured against him. The physician then refused to answer further questions regarding his malpractice case on the grounds of irrelevancy. The lower court denied a motion by the patient's counsel to compel the witness to answer further questions regarding the previous malpractice suit, and on appeal this ruling was upheld. The appellate court stated that the counsel either knew the answer to the question or questions regarding the previous malpractice suit, or could obtain it from the public record. It maintained that the only fact that he could discover would be a test of the witness' memory; therefore the appellate court confirmed the judgment of the lower court and stated that the witness had a right to be examined only as to relevant matter (Georgia Ct. of App., 3/2/71; *Cochran vs Neely*, 181 S.E. 2d 511. Rehearing denied 3/25/71).

Scheduling Appointments for Defendant Examinations

The receptionist should not schedule an excessive number of complicated defense examinations, especially those with thick files for review, for the same day, as they require a considerable amount of time and constitute a definite burden for the examining physician. It is preferable to limit this type to no more than two or three per day in order to provide time for private patients. In partnership or group practice, defendant examinations should be scheduled only for those physicians who are interested in performing such examinations.

A problem often arises when patients call and state they have been referred by their attorney. This may be true, but they do not state that the attorney has been instructed by the defendant's insurance company to have his client examined on their behalf. When the patient arrives, he or she may state that they were referred by their attorney (true) but make no mention of the insurance company, and the chart is processed as a plaintiff's case. This procedure requires the signing of assignment forms, and administration of treatment if indicated; however, for a defendant's examination neither of these would be expected. It is a good idea, therefore, to alert the receptionist to question the identity of the referring party—be it attorney or insurance company. Occasionally, this misrepresentation is done deliberately, by either the patient or his attorney, in an effort to obtain the best possible report from the defendant's physician. After the examiner has submitted his report to the plaintiff attorney, he cannot alter or add to that report even though the reports are returned to him with a notation that they should have been sent to the defendant (he can be sure the attorney has made photostatic copies and will produce them at trial if indicated).

In a group or partnership practice, if an appointment is made without the knowledge that it was for an insurance company and may involve court testimony, it may have been assigned to the wrong physician, as not all partners will be interested in these examinations. The referral may have been to one specific physician who customarily performs examinations for that company, and he may not be in the office that day. Usually most physicians will examine plaintiff cases, but often one specific physician has been requested to examine a plaintiff by the defendant carrier, and obviously the examination should be performed by that particular doctor. If the patient appears in the office and the selected examiner is not available, the patient may refuse to return, stating that the examination must be done that day, as he has taken leave from work, his time is too valuable to waste, and so on. In this situation the patient may demonstrate considerable hostility and resentment. In some instances the appointment can be arranged only with a court order, which is required in order to compel the patient to report for the examination.

One method of avoiding this complication is to compile a "Hold File," in which reports forwarded by the defendant are held until the patient appears for his appointment. When the patient is referred by an attorney unknown to the office, this file should be checked and it may identify the true source of the referral. In a busy office, with many phones ringing, this is not always possible at the time of the initial phone call from the patient requesting the medical appointment. However, the "Hold File" should always be checked when the patient appears, especially if the patient's attorney has not had any previous relationship with that office. Another clue will be the date of the accident; if it occurred several months or even years in the past, the examination is most likely on behalf of a defendant, unless the attorney has either written or phoned to indicate that this particular examination is being made for him in an effort to ascertain the true nature of his client's continued complaints. In some instances the patient may have been unhappy with his previous medical treatment, or his lawyer may desire a more comprehensive medical evaluation by a specialist before proceeding with settlement discussions or filing suit.

A capable physician who performs competent and fair examinations and writes a satisfactory medical report will soon receive many requests from insurance companies and defendant attorneys for his services. Unfortunately there are only a few physicians who are able to give good testimony and prepare proper medico-legal reports and these physicians soon find themselves greatly in demand by many insurance carriers. As a result, the doctor's private practice may suffer from excessive use of his available appointment time for defendant examinations; it is particularly irritating when these patients fail to show for their appointments and other patients have been refused.

As the number of defendant examinations increases, so too will the number of alerts for trial, necessitating an increasing scheduling of out-of-the-office time for that purpose. Inasmuch as a great majority of these cases are settled before trial, most of these alerts will not require the doctor's presence at court. However, in most instances the settlement or postponement of trial does not occur until from twenty-four to forty-eight hours before trial, and in some cases is announced on the day of trial.

Court commitments result in a severe encroachment upon the doctor's appointment and surgical schedule and other activities. Should he have six to eight alerts a week in several court jurisdictions, such as the District of Columbia, Virginia, and Maryland, or several on the same day, he is severely handicapped in his clinical practice. Most insurance companies and defendant attorneys recognize the imposition and demands on the doctor's professional schedule, and provide some compensation for cancelled appointment time so that he can be available to testify. However, this is usually not the full fee for testimony and does not adequately compensate him for the time lost from his practice.

Ultimately, the doctor must make a decision whether or not to limit the medico-legal portion of his practice, particularly if he has an active clinical practice. Ironically, should he desire to restrict it and specialize in medico-legal evaluations, this will limit the effectiveness of his testimony, as the plaintiff attorneys will point out in cross-examination that he is a "professional type of witness." Paradoxically, a doctor who has a large clinical practice and uses only a minor percentage of his time for defendant examinations, has more prestige and more stature in court.

In some jurisdictions, such as the District of Columbia, the court calendar is crowded and trial rarely starts on the day for which it is alerted. In many instances, the witnesses, attorneys, and litigants must wait on a day-to-day alert, sometimes for a week or more. Obviously, it is impossible for a doctor to have a full office schedule and still be available to testify on an hour's notice as some attorneys suggest. Fortunately, in most jurisdictions a definite trial date can be given and the doctor's time can be pinpointed fairly effectively to a morning or afternoon of that day. Measures are currently being taken to establish a firm trial date in the District of Columbia similar to the practice in Virginia and Maryland.

If the doctor performs a great number of defendant's examinations for a large insurance carrier or legal firm, the latter may refuse to pay for missed appointments or cancelled time for testimony, on the grounds that the large volume of business more than compensates the doctor for his lost time, hardly a fair solution. This may lead to strained relations, whereas a cooperative and cordial relationship is most desirable and should be worth the small additional cost to the defendant. A cooperative, competent physician is of great value to an insurance carrier, but a doctor who feels that his professional time is being wasted without compensation will perform his evaluations with diminished enthusiasm. The doctor must never put himself in a position where the defendant feels that he can control or dictate the type of report he desires. He should continue to treat plaintiffs as well as to examine defendants, in order to preserve his neutral status.

DIAGNOSIS

After a complete examination the examiner should be prepared to make a definite diagnosis without hedging. The diagnoses should be enumerated in order of importance and clearly stated; a narrative statement regarding the injuries is indefinite, possibly obscure, and generally not satisfactory. Standard accepted nomenclature, such as is used in the military services and has been adopted by medical librarians, should be employed for each diagnosis. Ranges and degrees of motion should follow the standard pattern as stated by the American Academy of Orthopaedic Surgeons, which has formulated a table for each joint. Terms such as *acute* and *chronic* should be used correctly and discussed if there is any variance or unusual factor; *minimal, mild, moderate,* and *severe* should be used where indicated to point out the degree of severity of the injury or disability. The doctor may wish to discuss the significance of *positive* tests which help to sustain his diagnosis, but he should also indicate clearly the significance of *normal* physical findings and *negative* tests. A well-stated opinion will help to prepare the attorney for trial and also facilitate settlement discussions.

Interpretation of Clinical Findings

The interpretation of his physical and x-ray examinations may pose a difficult problem for the physician. He must confine himself to the facts, and he is not permitted to interpret a medico-legal case in the same manner as a private case; in the medico-legal case he is subject to cross-examination and he must be able to sustain his opinions on the witness stand. Unfortunately, many of the findings are a matter of subjective interpretation and are not mathematically indisputable. This aspect can be minimized if the doctor uses all possible objective aids to augment the basis for his diagnosis and prognosis (Figure 10).

The evaluation of drugs in the relief of pain must take into account the wide variation in sensitivity and threshold of pain among various individuals. A nervous patient is apt to react less favorably to the same dosage of a narcotic or analgesic than a patient with a higher threshold of pain. Larger doses of analgesics are required for nervous individuals, often combined with adequate tranquilizing drugs. If a patient's history reflects prolonged use of strong analgesic and tranquilizing drugs without symptomatic relief, it may reflect a functional basis for his recurrent problems, particularly if the physical examination is unremarkable.

Anxiety states may be identified, but positive psychiatric diagnosis should be avoided. Qualifying statements should describe residuals of injury, such as moderate limitation of joint motion, secondary muscle atrophy, fractures healed with angulation or shortening, etc. Any discovered non-surgical condition which is related to the accident, should be stated; if the association is uncertain, it may be qualified as *possibly* or *probably* "due to trauma." Any pre-existing condition which is present should be noted as such, but a statement may be made regarding possible traumatic aggravation. In individuals with bizarre complaints frequently a detailed and meticulous examination will

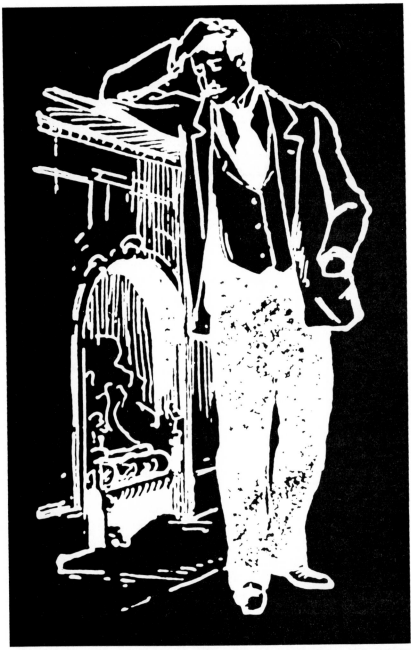

FIGURE 10. THE PHYSICIAN MUST BE ASTUTE. USE ALL YOUR
FACULTIES!

reveal evidence of the true nature of their complaints. An individual who continues to complain of her neck or lower back, yet has not had any medical attention for months even though it is readily available to her, probably has either psychosomatic or feigned symptoms rather than residuals of organic injury. For example, a bookkeeper at a hospital continued to complain of pain down her left hand, tracing it along the path of the ulnar nerve to the 4th and 5th fingers. She had received a few weeks of traction therapy, with benefit, three years before the examination but no further treatment. Treatment was readily available to her, and her treating physician encountered her constantly at the hospital; yet she was examined by him on only two occasions, ten months before and just prior to the defendant's examination. Obviously, if she had complained to her physician in the same manner that she complained to the defendant examiner, he would have ordered more physical therapy, including traction to her neck, to alleviate the alleged radicular pain. On clinical testing she complained of numbness in the entire 4th and 5th fingers, not following the anatomical 1½ finger pattern; in addition, she had glove-type hypesthesia of the left forearm which was definitely functional in origin. This case illustrates that a detailed history and careful evaluation of all factors is necessary to form a correct interpretation in a medico-legal case.

Patients will frequently manifest more symptoms to the defendant's physician than to their own physician whom they may have seen only a few days before, in an effort to impress the former with their alleged disabilities. Patients with back pain complain of inability to do housework, bend, stoop, and so forth, yet have regular marital relations. Recently an x-ray of the lumbosacral spine made of such an individual revealed a contraceptive diaphragm in place. She may have had pain with her housework but apparently this did not interfere with her marital chores!

If no objective clinical or x-ray evidence is found to substantiate the patient's continued subjective complaints, a statement should be made to this effect. The diagnosis should be factual and not a result of the examiner's suspicions based on the patient's complaints. The physician should not make a definite diagnosis on the basis of subjective symptoms alone as he can be misled by exaggeration. If he is not certain about a particular portion of the examination, he should so state and not make a firm statement which may be erroneous. The defendant examiner should remember that he is examining a claimant, not a patient seeking treatment, and frequently the symptoms recited are self-serving declarations which emphasize his claim rather than his desire for a cure. However this should not be interpreted to assume that all plaintiffs are dishonest. The examiner should always begin his examination with a fair and impartial attitude, but be wary of unsubstantiated complaints. The treating physician must be certain he can substantiate his diagnosis in court; otherwise a clever cross-examiner may cause him considerable humiliation.

Functional Symptoms

In acute low back disorders, the symptoms should be evaluated whether they are functional or organic in nature. The term *functional* implies that the complaint is predominantly an emotional adaptation which may be provoked by environmental factors, whereas the word *organic* indicates a definite structural change in an anatomical part. Sullivan states that evaluation of a functional disorder should include the following points: whether the patient's symptoms are consistent with organic disease and the total clinical picture, circumstances of onset, including emotional and interpersonal factors, significance patient attaches to his symptoms, advantages gained by his symptoms, and consistency of the symptom with a psychiatric illness.[34]

The most frequent psychosomatic phenomenon is the persistence of disease over a long period, coupled with the failure to respond to correct and adequate treatment. The patient may receive treatment of various modalities, including physical therapy, steroid injections, nerve blocks, immobilization, exercises, varied medications, and so on, but none is successful in relieving his symptoms. He may admit to temporary improvement for a few hours or perhaps a day after a therapy session, but he returns to the doctor with persistent symptoms unchanged in intensity or nature. An astute physician should recognize the probability of a strong psychosomatic factor in this type of patient, one who may continue under medical care for several months or even years; the emotional element becomes more apparent when complaints are unaltered by proper medication or environmental change and all indicated tests and studies are performed with negative results. These cases are more likely to be of psychosomatic origin than a result of organic disease or injury.[6]

Few cases of medical or surgical illness remain absolutely unchanged for several years, particularly when the patient has been adequately studied and treated. Most diseases are either progressive or regressive and do not remain *status quo* for prolonged periods of time. Defendant examiners are frequently faced with evaluating the patients of competent physicians who, even after many months or even years, have failed to recognize the strong psychosomatic factors producing their patient's persistent subjective complaints. The individual who fails to respond to correct treatment despite intensive efforts by his physician, soon becomes a disturbing visitor to the office and usually continues to return periodically until his case is resolved. Recognition and proper treatment of these difficult clinical problems in a reasonable period of time would facilitate settlement and a fair resolution of medico-legal cases which otherwise develop into bitterly contested litigation.

Evaluation of Pain

Evaluation of pain may be difficult, especially in a case where the proclamation of pain may be self-serving, such as a medico-legal case. At a recent joint meeting sponsored by the American Medical Association and the American Bar Association, Dr. Harold Williams of San Francisco called the refusal of physicians or lawyers to believe a person who says he is in pain, one of the saddest testimonials of cynicism within the two professions. He stated that a litigant's complaints should be given the same degree of credence as those of any patient, and the physician should exercise all the medical curiosity he can muster to ascertain the true nature and cause of the complaints.[36]

An indirect measure of the degree of pain may be inferred from the pattern of use of narcotic and analgesic drugs. If the patient states he still has quite a few pills left from his initial prescription for an analgesic or muscle relaxant, but still complains of continuing discomfort, the doctor should refer to his initial prescription. (It is a good idea to keep a carbon copy of all prescriptions given, particularly in medico-legal cases.) If it is noted that, had the patient taken the medication as prescribed, he should have exhausted his supply, there is some doubt as to the amount of actual pain that he had been suffering during this period. If refills were authorized, the doctor should always note on his records when a refill has been authorized over the phone with the pharmacist. Another indication of this inattention to medication may be the patient's inability to repeat the exact dosage schedule prescribed, as obviously had he been taking the pills regularly he would be familiar with the dosage.

Pain is a strange and complex phenomenon that often defies description. Some pains originate in the mind, and others in the body. Can a person tell the difference between a purely physical pain, and a psychosomatic pain—that is, pain which is triggered by mental or emotional problems, as fear, worry, and anxiety?

Careful studies of physical pain and psychosomatic pain provide a clue which may help individuals determine which type of pain they may be feeling at any given time. Physical pain tends to be intermittent and varying. Psychosomatic pain tends to be continuous and unvarying. It is the kind of pain which persists and remains constant with the person.

Even with these clues, it is not always possible to tell whether pain stems from the mind, or from the body. Often there may be a vexing combination of both mental and physical symptoms.

It is easy to become anxious and alarmed when we have a pain, and to wonder if it is a symptom of something serious. The cure for this anxiety is to have the doctor check it out to determine whether it is physical or otherwise. Studies show, however, that a great many of our every-day aches and pains are very definitely affected by our mental and emotional attitudes.

Evaluation of the psychological factors and their effect on the production of symptoms requires experience, competence, and awareness on the part of the examining physician. In most instances, a psychiatrist is not employed, and the conclusions must be made by the examining physician based on his own personal experiences and professional observations. A. J. Enelow,[7] Professor of Psychiatry at the University of Southern California, insists that physicians must give increased attention to the complexity surrounding the whole problem of compensable injury. A personal injury that makes a person eligible for compensation is usually complicated by emotional problems, particularly after encounters with insurance agents, attorneys, claims agents, labor union representatives, judges, hearing examiners and others. The psychological factors add to the difficulty and jeopardize his motivation for full recovery.

Dr. Enelow states that such factors are twice as frequent in Workmen's Compensation injuries as in those which are not compensable injuries. He indicates that individuals most likely to develop psychiatric complications after injury are the hysterical patient, the dependent and immature patient, the overconscientious worker who is incapable of accepting help and tries to resolve his conflict by overwork, the depressed patient who may have a suicidal tendency, and the sociopathic exploiter who has self-seeking values in an attempt to circumvent a society which he considers an adversary. This is the individual who has constant conflicts with authority, frequently changes jobs and attempts to manipulate others to his own advantage. It is in this sociopathic group that malingering is most common. An individual without psychiatric complications, particularly where there is no compensation element, will accept help from others but immediately discard his dependent state when he is able to resume normal activities.

It is universally recognized that the present system of compensation associated with Workmen's Compensation illness or accident may aggravate the problem of returning the patient to work, especially where there is a functional or emotional element. When the patient consults an attorney immediately after the injury or shortly after undergoing treatment, the physician may become

suspicious of his true motivation, as there is no need for the help
of an attorney if there has been a compensable accident. The
Workmen's Compensation law provides adequate guarantee for
treatment and payment for disability; the law is designed to
protect the employee more than the employer. In addition, the
Workmen's Compensation commissioner will make every effort
to protect the employee with or without an attorney. If he consults an attorney before or soon after consulting a physician, there
may be doubt as to the real nature of his injury, particularly if
there are no objective findings. This is particularly true if the
patient's history includes a past incident where he has had legal
representation as the result of a minor injury. Sometimes, however,
the patient has been referred to a lawyer by his union representative and is merely following orders; he should not be faulted
for that, particularly if he is not intelligent or knowledgeable
on compensation rights.

Patients with joint pain that has been aggravated by injury,
particularly male patients, may have gout. It has long been known
that trauma will activate dormant gout with resultant hyper-
uricemia and clinical manifestations. The examiner should be
suspicious of gout where there is evidence of soft tissue swelling,
tenderness, painful and limited motion, joint effusion, and
synovial thickening, particularly in the knee or elbow following
an accident. A blood uric acid and a careful history of preceding
joint problems will be helpful in establishing a diagnosis. Gout
is more prevalent than generally recognized and is often present
for years without the patient's knowledge. An accidental injury
may trigger the condition into a recognizable entity which can
be controlled with proper treatment.

Physicians who examine or treat a large percentage of patients
involved in accidents with medico-legal ramifications frequently
note a high percentage of cervical injuries in women, particularly
in large metropolitan areas. Shutt and Dohan made a survey of
neck injuries to women in auto accidents, finding a ratio of 6.7
to 1000 women per year, about half from rear end collisions.
They believe that most of these could have been prevented by
properly designed headrests on the front seats to prevent the

initial sharp retroflexion of the neck following a rear impact with a forward propulsion of the car. Their findings did not support the popular opinion that the symptoms of "whiplash injury" are often due to the malingering and subconscious psychoneurotic mechanisms in an individual seeking monetary gain. They found that when disability occurred after a delayed onset it did not result in a longer period of disability than the disability of immediate onset. Although the intensity of complaints often increases after the patient has employed an attorney, this is not always true.[32]

The patient usually seeks medical attention promptly if he has been injured, before he goes to an attorney; however, the fact that a patient has consulted an attorney within a few days of the accident, before reporting to a doctor, should not be construed to indicate that he has had no real injury. He may be confused or may have sought the advice of an attorney for referral to a competent physician; in many instances he is more concerned about the large property damage to his car and getting his car back in operation, and pays little or no attention to the aches and pains of his body. When the pain continues after he has made arrangements for repair of his car, he then seeks medical attention.

Evaluation of Electroencephalogram

Electroencephalograms provide significant information after a head injury, particularly when they are repeated over an extended period of time. An abnormality which is present initially and disappears on subsequent studies most likely represents an injury related to the accident; it also demonstrates improvement and good progress. However, the persistence of an abnormality does not necessarily imply that permanent injury has been sustained. The interpretation of electroencephalograms is complicated and is dependent on the subjective interpretation and experience of the reporting physician; it is not a mere mathematical analysis. This variable can be eliminated if the electroencephalograms are repeated in the same laboratory and interpreted by the same physician.

It has been reported that about 10 to 12 per cent of all

"normal people" show some degree of abnormality without any history of any previous injuries or neurological difficulty. This was clearly demonstrated in a patient who was treated for head and neck injuries sustained in an automobile accident and referred to a neurosurgeon ten days after the accident. The first EEG tracing (dated 11-25-67) showed a mild abnormality. However, the patient had improved considerably in the interim and her headaches were much less frequent and considerably milder than at the previous reading, despite the persistence of the EEG abnormality. The neurologist concluded that the headaches had resulted from the accident but would not require further treatment. His report stated that an EEG abnormality resulting from a head injury usually can be expected to improve in a period of a few weeks or months, with the maximum abnormality expected shortly after the injury. If the EEG abnormality persists, then there is a possibility that the abnormality had been present before the date of injury. In this case, the EEG was repeated five months after the injury and showed no change; it was concluded that the abnormality was not related to the accident of November 1967. Further investigation revealed that the patient had suffered migraine headaches after giving birth several years before the accident, and had been treated with specific headache remedies over a period of several years with relief. This would explain the electroencephalogram pattern discovered after the accident.

Electroencephalograms have a definite value in diagnosis, but each individual case must be studied and a full history secured in order to properly evaluate any abnormality. Neurologists usually perform a series of electroencephalograms over an extended period of time whenever a deviation is discovered, in order to eliminate pre-existing abnormalities and provide a firm basis for their opinions and conclusions.

Malingering

After a negative physical examination in which there are insufficient objective findings to account for the patient's persistent subjective complaints, the examining physician must differentiate between voluntary and involuntary exaggeration of symptoms, malingering, and hysteria, in order to make an accurate diagnosis and prognosis and to institute proper treatment. Fortunately, true malingering is rare but exaggeration of symptoms is frequently encountered in a busy practice. It may be recognized by astute observation: various signs will aid in the differential diagnosis.

A true malingerer is one who actually feigns illness where none exists, whereas an individual who is exaggerating wishes his condition to appear more disabling and serious than it actually is; he enlarges upon the truth and magnifies his complaints. Hysteria is a form of psychoneurosis and represents a true mental illness, one which can be detected by careful observation and psychiatric investigation.

A definitive statement of malingering is difficult to substantiate without an exhaustive investigation. It is preferable to note the possibility or probability of malingering rather than a clear-cut statement. A useful phrase that the author has frequently employed in describing an individual who is obviously exaggerating his complaints is, "The patient appears to be voluntarily promoting his complaints."

The detection of the malingerer (or the individual with purposeful exaggeration) begins with the history, which is often vague, non-specific or prefaced with such remarks as, "I don't remember," "I didn't bring my notes with me," "Ask my attorney," "Ask my treating physician," or, "I just came here for a physical examination and you're not supposed to ask me any questions."

Such a patient will be vague and will not give exact details about the accident or his past history. If the examiner has been briefed with complete medical reports describing previous accidents or injuries which the patient does not reveal, he should certainly suspect this person's veracity. James Frenkil,[11] who has been actively engaged in practice related to occupational diseases for many years, sometimes refers to an insurance index bureau for detailed history of previous claims, or even checks on personal health and accident claims through the patient's insurance coverage.

Another clue may be the source of referral of the patient. If the patient did not see a physician after the injury, but first consulted his lawyer, then a doctor, it would appear that his injury was relatively minor (but not always!) If he has a past history of similar claims with legal representation for each minor injury, this too would raise the index of suspicion. History of repeated injuries to the same area after minor accidents, followed by long periods of treatment and legal representation, should merit thorough investigation and observation.

The doctor should also be wary of the patient who has had a second accident before he recovers from the first, and states that the first accident involved his lower back, the second his neck, and neither of the areas was affected by the separate accidents. Obviously he is promoting two separate claims. If he already had a severe backache, for example, then had another accident serious enough to cause a moderately severe injury to his neck, in all likelihood there would be some aggravation to his low back condition along with the neck injury, but the claims-conscious patient will try to keep the two injuries apart.

The patient who is not being frank with his treating physician may state that he never had any previous difficulty with the affected area, such as the neck, prior to the accident, even though x-rays taken on the day of the accident revealed advanced osteoarthritis which must have limited neck motion. The patient who denies any earlier problem does not wish to jeopardize his present claim, whereas a truthful patient will usually admit some pre-existing difficulty which was relatively minor until the accident; this pattern is characteristic of traumatic aggravation of a prior condition. Males may claim that the accident prevents normal sex relationships, in an attempt to explain diminished sex ability; older people may claim that the accident caused such symptoms as blurred vision, high blood pressure, arthritis, kidney problems, etc. To mention only one, the complaint of blurred or diminished vision is quite prevalent but is rarely substantiated by ophthalmologic examination, which frequently reveals a refractory error unrelated to trauma.

Finally, malingering, or gross exaggeration of symptoms, is

likely to be found in the patient who makes frequent switches from one doctor to another, or from one physical therapist to another, complaining about inadequate treatment or lack of attention. The examiner should suspect the patient who, in response to queries, constantly refers to his lawyer and who seems to be more concerned about the legal ramifications of his case than about a medical cure for his ills.

Orthopaedic Examination of the Malingerer

Examination begins with observation in the waiting room as well as in the examining room. If the patient is observed to be sitting comfortably while waiting to be called, then walks without difficulty into the examining room and quickly undresses, whereupon, in the presence of the examiner, he manifests an unusual amount of discomfort and an inability to move about the room or to ascend the examining table—the examining physician should certainly be alerted to probable exaggeration or malingering.

In his examination of the cervical spine, the doctor should note the ease with which the patient turns his head to either side for inspection of his ears; also the way he tilts his head into extension for examination of the nose and throat (i.e. with tongue depressor); or the ease with which he turns his head to either side to avoid breathing on the examiner during the chest examination. All of these signs should be *casually* observed but *carefully noted* by the doctor. If the patient stiffens and refuses to move his head and neck when he measures the range of cervical motion with the Cervigon Protractor in contrast to the easy motion exhibited for the ENT and chest examination, this is an obvious signal of gross exaggeration.

There are several testing procedures which have been developed to ascertain the authenticity of the patient's complaints. One such test is to have the patient stand erect, abduct the shoulders to 90 degrees, flex the elbows and make a tight fist with the examiner grasping the patient's hands. He is asked whether this produces any pain or discomfort in the scapular or cervical region; if the patient answers affirmatively, it is obvious that he is exaggerating as there is no anatomical association.

Another excellent test involves the Jamar dynamometer, described on pp. 38–41 under "Grip Testing," which permits an accurate estimate of the patient's gripping power. By using the apparatus with different grip openings, then repeating after a rest interval of five minutes, the patient's veracity can be checked, as the readings show no more than a 10 per cent variance for each opening if maximum effort has been exerted on each testing. (See Figure 4).

Sensory testing which reveals bizarre hypesthesia patterns may provide an excellent clue to the type of individual being examined. If the patient reports a stocking or glove type of hypesthesia of the arms or legs, completely involving the entire extremity or limited to above or below the elbows or knees, or demonstrating hemianaesthesia of one half of his body without paralysis or serious cranial or spinal lesions, this would definitely present a non-organic condition. Vibratory sensation should be tested with a tuning fork and is of special value as it is impaired only when there has been injury to the postero-lateral spino-thalamic tract by a major brain stem or cerebellar lesion, such as a large hemorrhage or brain tumor, which would be grossly obvious if present. Patients who have had several examinations in the past may have studied the response to pin prick testing, but very few are aware of the significance of tuning fork testing.

Detection of low back fraud has been discussed by many observers, and many tests have been devised to aid in diagnosis. Objective findings are singularly important. True muscle spasm is objective if it is persistent and not intermittent in nature. The patient who has muscle spasm in his back and holds himself rigidly, but when observed a few moments later moves his back freely, is exercising voluntary control. Spasm after a back sprain is constant and often produces spastic scoliosis; it continues without change, particularly when the patient is erect. Sometimes the muscles relax when the patient lies prone and removes the effect of gravity, but this is a normal physiological response. If the lumbar lordotic curve reverses and disappears as the back is flexed forward, this is not consistent with involuntary muscle spasm; with true muscle spasm the curve does not flatten or reverse itself, there is limited back flexion, and the deformity persists.

A number of authors have noted the following method of detecting the true amount of back flexion. The patient who is unable to flex his back forward even a few degrees while standing is placed on the examining table with his knees fully extended; if he has no organic block to flexing his hips and bending forward, he can flex his back easily past 90 degrees and sometimes reach his fingertips to his toes. He does not realize that he has now flexed his back in the same manner as if he were in the erect position. Another variation of this test is to have the patient sit on the examining table, place his outstretched legs on a chair and then sit up straight, again demonstrating good back flexion. A few examiners have tried having the patient kneel on a chair, and then flex forward to touch his fingertips to the floor; this is a difficult maneuver to perform and the author has not found it useful as most patients will not cooperate in this test.

Tenderness should be localized, not vague, and should be consistently noted, whether or not the patient's attention is diverted by speech or simultaneous palpation elsewhere. If the patient withdraws with light touch over an allegedly tender area, yet a moment later allows you to press quite firmly in the same area while distracting him with conversation and palpation of a more distant area with the other hand, this is not true tenderness and it is being feigned. A patient with a severely sprained ankle will complain and withdraw from pressure over the sprained area whether or not his attention is diverted. Packard[30] mentions the patient who will knock the physician's hand away, or grab the physician's hand as he tries to palpate the area, because it is too painful to touch. This observation, coupled with others, is a signal to arouse suspicion in the examiner, who should then perform other tests to verify his tentative diagnosis of exaggeration or malingering.

We have had occasion to refer to another type—the female patient who comes into the office wearing a collar and holding her neck very stiffly, yet is exquisitely dressed with long earrings, extensive eye make-up, fashionable hairdo and a long zipper in the back of her blouse. This patient may display gross disability and apparent intensive discomfort, which is usually exaggerated as the patient in acute pain ordinarily is not so painstaking in her appearance.

In the patient who is faking, manual testing of strength in the upper or lower extremities may manifest apparent marked weakness, despite good muscle tone and the lack of measurable or visible muscle atrophy.

In low back syndromes the patient who points to the bony prominence of the mid or lower sacrum as the site of his discomfort should immediately arouse suspicions, as this is not a site of musculo-ligamentous strain; the patient may allege exquisite tenderness over the bony sacral prominence but no tenderness over the lumbosacral joint or the paravertebral area at L-4-5, where ligamentous pathology usually occurs.

A useful test for low back pain that the author first proposed in a scientific exhibit in 1963 is performed with the patient lying face down on the examining table, knees flexed 90 degrees. The patient is asked to flex his toes against resistance with the examiner holding his toes; he is asked whether this produces any pain in his back or neck, and this is then repeated with toe extension. If the patient alleges pain in the lumbar or dorsal region, it is obvious that this is not true pain as there is no anatomical association between the maneuver performed and the alleged discomfort. After performing this test, some patients will put on a real exhibition of discomfort, yelling and grimacing with alleged pain, trying to crawl off the table; they continue to complain of pain after this maneuver, stating that the doctor has caused them great damage and injury as a result of this test. Of course, here again is excellent corroboration of the doctor's suspicions that he is dealing with malingering or at least gross exaggeration.

Some doctors have resorted to the possibly unfair pretext of having their nurse walk in on a male patient with his pants down and observing his quick protective reaction. Observation of the patient without his knowledge is always useful; this can be done by observing the patient's gait and activities after he leaves by looking through the window or following him down the hall. The limp that immediately clears up after leaving the office is of course a fake one. In one instance, the author observed a man who had been limping about the office in gross discomfort, running to catch a cab that was about to leave the driveway. A one-way mirror can be utilized to make undetected observations but may not be considered ethical medical practice; the doctor may be placed in a difficult position when giving such testimony in court.

Full Disclosure of all Diagnoses and Objective Findings

In an examination for the defense, the examiner should provide the information requested, and generally not involve himself in other areas of the body which are diseased or injured but have no causal relationship with the accident in question. However, he should briefly note all pathology discovered during the examination, for future reference; his doing so will indicate that the examiner was observant, astute, and thorough (Figure 10). The completeness of his examination may save embarrassment in cross-questioning by opposing counsel, who often tries to depreciate the expert testimony through insignificant details not associated with the accident being litigated. In addition, the defendant will be in a better position to refute a belated claim trying to associate these defects with the litigation. Some examples are deformities of poliomyelitis, old scars, foot deformities, old fracture deformities, residuals of stroke such as paralysis, and so on.

All diagnoses should be reported whether or not they are helpful to the party employing his services. If the examiner finds a condition adverse to the party for whom he is making the examination, he should definitely include that diagnosis in his report but without any discussion. He may be asked to elaborate at a later date, at which time he should make a truthful and factual presentation; in his initial report this is not required and may hinder a successful settlement of the suit. For example, if a defendant examiner finds evidence of arthritis, this should be reported, but it is not necessary to state that the patient's continuing symptoms are probably due to activation of a previously dormant arthritic condition, and that the aggravated arthritis condition may persist indefinitely; this is beyond the demands of a defense examination.

Should the defendant examiner discover a fracture that had been missed by the treating physician, he should note the fracture in his report and discuss the effect of this untreated fracture on the patient's present condition. Such a discovery may explain the patient's continued complaints and lack of progress. Under these conditions the defendant examiner should contact the treating physician, either by phone or by mailing him a copy of his report, and refer the patient back to him for further treatment. There should be no detailed discussion with the patient, and he should exercise every care to avoid any derogatory comment about the treatment or missed diagnosis. He should also suggest that the patient be referred back to him for re-examination after the fracture has been adequately treated, so that he may make a final evaluation after the patient has received the maximum benefit of medical care.

Where arthritic changes have developed after any injury to a joint, such as the knee, he should report the x-ray presence of the arthritic changes. If the examiner feels secure in making a diagnosis of post-traumatic arthritis, he should do so, but if he believes the degenerative changes could represent progressive osteoarthritis, then he should describe the changes noted without making a definitive diagnosis. A sharp attorney will understand the description and use the facts accordingly. On the other hand if a diagnosis of post-traumatic arthritis is made, and it later becomes evident that this is not true, then settlement will be delayed, as the demand for recovery by the plaintiff will be greatly increased by the erroneous diagnosis and resultant probability of permanent difficulty and need of further medical care.

Specific disability ratings should never be stated when making an examination for the defendant unless they are particularly requested. For example, if the treating physician for the plaintiff has made such a rating, then the defendant examiner may be requested to comment on that figure and state his opinion. Usually, however, no ratings are stated by the treating physician; a disability rating volunteered by the defendant examiner could be strong evidence for the plaintiff, interfering with settlement proceedings and resulting in a trial which could have been avoided. This is of particular importance if the defendant physician performs frequent examinations and continues to make the same error; he will then be losing a considerable amount of his valuable professional time in court.

Disability ratings ordinarily should not be based only on the patient's history and subjective complaints, where there is complete lack of objective findings by clinical or x-ray examination. It should be noted that the patient's declarations are "self-serving" in interest. Frequently the examiner is impressed with the integrity of the patient but, in the absence of confirming clinical signs, he cannot with assurance state that a definite disability exists. In some incidences, a history which recounts all details of the accident and subsequent treatment will disclose obvious discrepancies, resulting in skepticism as to the patient's veracity. Most physicians recognize that a patient may have a few vague complaints which are difficult to corroborate by clinical examination, but on the other hand, the high incidence of nervous tension which produces subjective complaints is well established. Several texts have been written on this very subject. Individuals who appear to be quite stable may still manifest nervous tension under the stress of work problems and domestic conflicts, with resultant vague subjective complaints after an injury or accident. Thus a disability rating based on subjective complaints is not realistic and cannot be substantiated. It is better to note the presence of subjective complaints and record the lack of any objective signs, then state the examiner's impression of the integrity and cooperation of the patient. This will leave *the door ajar* and give a fair representation of the facts. The examiner may have another opportunity to re-examine the patient and amplify or verify his initial impressions.

3 TREATMENT

Patients involved in accidents with medico-legal aspects should be treated in the same manner as any other type of patient. Treatment should be directed toward restoring the patient to an active working status as quickly as possible, utilizing all modalities of therapy which are indicated for each individual case.

MEDICATION AND DUPLICATE PRESCRIPTIONS

A muscle relaxant or analgesic drug is usually prescribed to relieve the distress accompanying a musculo-ligamentous strain or sprain. Adequate tranquilizing medication should be provided for the apprehensive patient with a nervous reaction; this may be obvious or expressed by fear of traveling in motor vehicles, recurrent frightening dreams, or speculation about the accident in which he was involved, such as "I constantly think how miraculous it was that I wasn't killed." The dosage and selection of the tranquilizing drug should be adjusted to the patient's status and need; inquiry should be made whether or not he has used tranquilizers before, whether he will be driving a vehicle since his perceptive faculties may be diminished by the resultant tranquilizing effect, and whether the patient is working as the drug may jeopardize his working activities. The patient should be warned of possible side effects and advised to reduce the dosage if there are any adverse reactions from the tranquilizer drug.

Headache is a frequent complaint after many types of accidents, even though the major injuries are elsewhere. The severity varies with the nervous temperament of the patient, and whether, for instance, there is a past history of headaches such as migraine.

The doctor should inquire regarding previous headache remedies before prescribing specific medication. In all instances a carbon copy of the prescription should be securely attached to the chart for future reference and accurate record. Carbon paper should be inserted in the prescription pad routinely as a duplicate may be very valuable if a problem arises later.

Occasionally a female patient (Males too!) will return to the office and state that she continues to have the same difficulties, such as pain in the lower back as on her initial visit. Examination reveals definite nervousness and anxiety. When questioned about the prescription for a tranquilizer which had been ordered on the first visit, she may deny that she ever received one or, as one patient stated, "You gave one to my husband (also a patient), not to me." A duplicate prescription stapled to her clinical record will immediately demonstrate to the patient that she has been un-cooperative, and her complaints usually become less vociferous. Such an event indicates the type of individual under care and the doctor should be skeptical of additional complaints.

PHYSICAL THERAPY

Physical therapy is a useful aid to relieve pain and swelling from musculo-ligamentous injuries and helps restore the injured part to full function. It should not be prescribed indiscriminately; specific modalities should be ordered for the condition to be treated. For example, a cervical sprain usually responds to hydro-collator (hot packs), massage, and Sayre halter traction; ultra-sonic and medcosonlator therapy are also quite helpful. The amount of traction is gradually increased depending on the patient's reaction to this treatment; some patients are unable to tolerate traction as it increases their pain. Occasionally, patients react unfavorably to ultrasonic and electrical stimulation and this too must be stopped.

In the low back area, lumbar and lumbosacral sprains are usually helped by hot packs, massage, medcosonlator and ultra-sonic therapy, occasionally by diathermy; later back-strengthen-ing exercises such as the Williams routine are added when the pain subsides. Whirlpool baths, paraffin baths, hot packs and ultrasonic therapy often relieve the discomfort of hematomata, sprains, and injuries to the extremities such as severe contusions, tendinitis and bursitis (Figure 11).

After the initial examination, a card outlining the treatment schedule should be completed and sent with the patient to the physical therapist. This card provides an interim record until the patient's chart has been typed. It also informs the physical therapist when the patient should return to the doctor for a check-up examination.

PHYSICAL THERAPY TREATMENT SCHEDULE

DATE_____

NAME:

RECOMMENDED THERAPY:
> A. Areas to be treated
> B. Modalities
> C. Schedule of treatments

CHECK-UP EXAM:

DATES OF TREATMENT:

The frequency of physical therapy depends on the severity of the condition being treated. In most instances treatment is administered three times a week for the first two to three weeks, then twice a week, then once a week. In unusual circumstances, daily therapy may be indicated for the first week or so, but the doctor should weigh the inconvenience and discomfort of daily trips to the office against the positive value of frequent therapy, as some of the benefits may be dissipated by the daily auto rides to his office. If the patient is sufficiently injured to warrant daily physical therapy, it may be wiser to hospitalize the patient for a short period until his condition improves. This would provide the needed rest and intensive therapy without the disadvantage of frequent automobile trips and would accelerate his progress. Hospitalization is also indicated to provide leg or pelvic traction (for example, Buck's Extension Traction) for acute back strain or herniated disc syndrome (Figure 12).

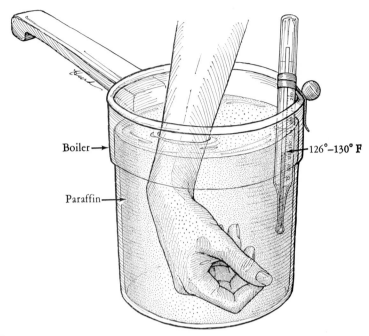

Boiler→

Paraffin—

126°–130° F

FIGURE 11. HOME PARAFFIN BATHS.

Useful to replace or supplement office therapy. Helpful in restoration of hand, wrist, and finger motion, also to reduce swelling of foot, ankle, wrist and hand.

HOME PARAFFIN TECHNIQUE: Ordinary paraffin (8 parts) is added to mineral oil (1 part) in a boiler and the mixture heated to 126 to 130 degrees F. The hand and wrist are repeatedly dipped into the paraffin after allowing each application to harden. A paraffin "glove" is formed which should be left on for 20 minutes and then removed. Approximately 5 to 8 dips are usually required. After paraffin hardens, wrap hand in bath towel to retain heat during the 20 minute waiting period.

In no instance should a patient be placed on a prolonged course of physical therapy without a check-up examination at least every ten to fourteen days. This is a relatively simple matter for the physician who has an office fully equipped for physical therapy, as a check-up examination can be arranged in conjunction with one of the scheduled therapy sessions. If the patient has been referred to a hospital facility or to an independent physical

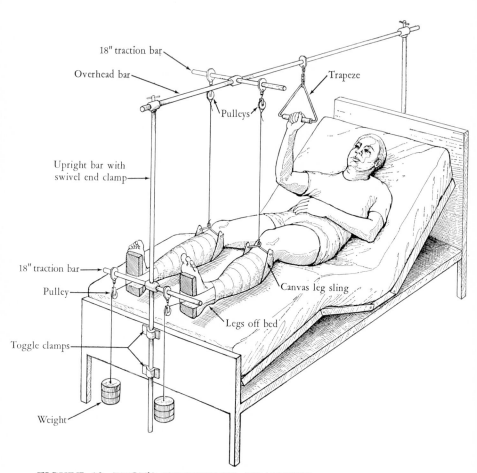

FIGURE 12. BUCK'S EXTENSION TRACTION.

A diagram prepared to instruct hospital personnel in the proper application of Buck's extension traction for maximum effect on the low back; designed to avoid friction with the bed covering. This type of traction has been effectively utilized by the author for many years, but pelvic traction may also be used. Without such a diagram, the leg traction with thigh slings is rarely applied correctly, unless hospital personnel have been working regularly with the treating physician.

therapist, then a check-up appointment for the physician should be made at regular intervals to determine the need for change in modality, frequency and duration of therapy. The decision should not be left to the physical therapist; however, if the patient is receiving treatment at a facility supervised by a physiatrist (a physician specializing in physical therapy), then the treatment program may be controlled by that physician.

In some instances nerve blocks may be indicated, but again this should not be performed indiscriminately. If the complaints constantly recur, then the blocks should be discontinued and not given indefinitely for a mere temporary effect.

Aspiration of fluids or blood from joints (arthrocentesis), such as from a knee joint, should be performed when indicated; hydrocortisone may be injected into the joint after aspiration. Elastic bandage supports, compression dressings, braces, crutches, canes, slings, etc. are used as required. Other injuries call for individual care according to the usual standards of medical practice, such as treatment of fractures, lacerations, abrasions, burns, and so on.

Consultation and specialized care should be requested if indicated, such as consultation with an ophthalmic surgeon, plastic surgery, neurosurgery, or even psychiatric help in occasional cases. In all instances, a record should be made of the treatment prescribed. This is usually included in the final paragraph of the medico-legal report. Accurate records regarding treatment are essential, not only for the reports but also for the protection of the doctor himself in the event of any possible future action against him for improper care.[18]

HOME CARE

A well-outlined plan of home treatment should accelerate the patient's progress. This ordinarily consists of dry or moist heat —warm showers or tub baths, or warm packs for extremity injuries, often followed by a rub with a liniment of the doctor's choice. One liniment found to be quite effective is made up of Chloroform 12 cc, Methyl-salicylate 48 cc, and Olive oil q.s. 120 cc. Paraffin baths for hand and wrist injuries or arthritis are often beneficial (Figure 11). Exercises for home use should be prescribed such as pendulum or Codman routine for shoulder muscles, exercises to increase the range of motion and strength of the neck, low back, knees, ankles, hips, elbows, wrists, fingers, and progressive resistance exercises (PRE) to improve muscle tone and strength.

Pamphlets are available for distribution entitled *Care of the Neck* and *Care of the Back,* which give the patient insight into his problems and graphically demonstrate the exercise routine, precautions in lifting, and give other helpful measures. These can be purchased at a nominal cost and used to supplement the doctor's oral instructions. In addition these pamphlets will give patients a written reference, as many are excited at the time of their office visit and misconstrue or forget oral instructions, thus slowing down their recovery. They are more apt to follow the doctor's advice if they can take home an instructive booklet.

PHYSICAL THERAPY AS AN AID IN DIAGNOSIS

The administration of a short treatment program may also have diagnostic value, particularly if it is difficult to accurately assess the extent of injury on the initial visit. Although an experienced examiner is usually able to make an accurate diagnosis on the first visit, there are times when the nervous element is so predominant that it obscures the organic pathology present. In such cases a short period of physical therapy will keep the patient under observation and give the doctor more foundation to diagnose his basic problems with less chance of having overlooked the correct diagnosis. After repeated exposure the physician will be able to differentiate the functional from the organic manifestations in such cases, but even the experienced physician can err. In cases of doubt it is wise to give two or three physical therapy treatments over a period of one to two weeks to insure an accurate diagnosis and prognosis. This is especially true when the patient is seen immediately after an accident, when he is often extremely nervous and emotionally upset.

However, once the doctor feels sure about the diagnosis and believes that there is no organic basis for the continued complaints, he should stop treatment and advise the patient accordingly. He should not continue to treat the patient indefinitely when he believes that the symptoms are largely psychosomatic in origin, as this only fixes the alleged disability in the patient's mind.

OFFICE TREATMENT AND EXERCISE FORMS

In a busy medical practice any hand-out memoranda is valuable if it will economize the doctor's time, such as explaining a treatment program. When first seen, the patient is usually in severe pain and distress and will not remember oral instructions. After the doctor has taken the time to explain the diagnosis and prognosis to the patient, he can hand him the needed instructions. Recommendations for treatment are frequently standard after such injuries as cervical and lumbosacral strain; a form can be devised which can be generally used, subject to occasional modification. This will enable the patient to follow instructions without omission or misinterpretation.

For the acute low back disorder there are several standard methods used in treatment which can be outlined in a separate memorandum. Exercises for the lower back are fairly standard; illustrated memorandum pads are distributed by various drug companies graphically showing the exercises and outlining precautions and instructions. The desired exercises can be checked and distributed to the patient. Cervical exercises are also fairly standard and can be similarly distributed.

Home care of acute low back disorders requires adherence to a strict regime to achieve good results. The following outline is useful as a handout; it may be modified as the treating physician desires.

Instructions for Home Care with Acute Low Back Disorder

1. Rest in bed with pillow under knees, one or two pillows under the head and shoulders; knees flexed and relaxed.

2. Bed board under mattress—½ to ¾ inch plywood for patient's half of the bed is sufficient.

3. Warm tub baths for 20 minutes, A.M. and P.M., putting 2 to 3 handfuls of crude epsom salts in the water.

4. Perform back exercises following tub baths, as instructed by physical therapist. Follow instruction sheet supplied by therapist.

5. Avoid any heavy lifting or straining. Remain off feet as much as possible.

6. Take medication as prescribed. If medication makes you sleepy, reduce pills (half dosage) following breakfast and lunch and take full dosage after dinner and at bedtime.

7. Report to the office for physical therapy as ordered. If unable to keep appointment, please notify in advance.

8. Use corset support (if prescribed) during the day; remove it at night.

9. Keep bowels loose, taking laxatives if necessary to avoid straining at stool; the straining will aggravate the back condition.

---

patient's name

---

doctor

To help ease your back pain:

BED Bed rest is advisable. If you must work, try to arrange rest periods during the working day. In any case, plan to spend more time in bed than you ordinarily would, retiring earlier and resting on weekends. Use a firm mattress!

BOARD A plywood board (¾ in. to 1 in. thick) should be placed directly under the mattress. This will help lessen the strain on your back. If boards are not available at department stores, a local lumber yard can cut one to order.

HEAT Moist heat is preferred. Relax in a hot bath, for twenty minutes, in the morning and evening.

At other times, apply hot towels to your back. Repeat these applications two to four times daily.

Special Instructions_____

FIGURE 13. "TO HELP EASE YOUR BACK PAIN."
Courtesy of A. H. Robins Company, Richmond, Va.

Brief instructions for home therapy for patients with acute low back strain, with emphasis on bed board and moist heat, are provided in the form entitled "To Help Ease Your Back Pain" (Figure 13). The form advises the patient how to obtain a bed board and also provides instruction regarding the use of moist heat.

Exercises for the low back are an essential part of any treatment program to relieve chronologically recurring pain in the dorso-lumbar spine. Exercise instruction sheets are available from several pharmaceutical firms. Few patients will retain all the oral instructions given on the initial visit; written instructions and diagrams are essential to a well supervised back exercise program. See "Exercises for Low Back Pain" (Figure 14).

Exercises to aid in the rehabilitation of a patient who has incurred an injury to the musculo-ligamentous structures of the neck are listed on the following form. They should be supplemented with verbal instructions and demonstrations of the exercises by either the doctor or his therapist.

Exercises for Cervical Strain

Stand under a hot shower for approximately 10-20 minutes and perform the following exercises (twice daily if possible):
1. Turn head slowly as far as possible to the right, then to the left.
2. Try to put chin on chest, slowly.
3. Raise head backward looking up at ceiling, slowly.
4. Try to touch left ear to the left shoulder.
5. Try to touch right ear to the right shoulder.
6. Raise both shoulders as close to the ears as possible and hold tightly for five counts and then carry shoulders backward as far as possible and hold tightly, then relax.
7. Stand on toes, hands clasped behind back (placed over buttocks), inhale, extend up toward ceiling, and pull downward and backward on shoulders throwing chest out, then exhale slowly.

Continue these exercises while under the shower but they can also be done during the day at odd moments. They will help relax and relieve tension of the neck and shoulder muscles.

Exercise programs to restore strength, range of motion, and improve function in the shoulder and knee are outlined in the

Exercises for low back pain

General Information:

Don't overdo exercising, especially in the beginning. Start by trying the movements slowly and carefully. Don't be alarmed if the exercises cause some mild discomfort which lasts a few minutes. But if pain is more than mild and lasts more than 15 or 20 minutes, *stop* and do no further exercises until you see your doctor.

Do the exercises on a hard surface covered with a thin mat or heavy blanket. Put a pillow under your neck if it makes you more comfortable. Always start your exercises slowly—and in the order marked—to allow muscles to loosen up gradually. Heat treatments just before you start can help relax tight muscles. Follow the instructions carefully; it will be well worth the effort.

Do exercises marked (**X**)

in numerical order

for _____ minutes

_____ times a day.

Take the medication

prescribed for you

_____ times daily

for_____.

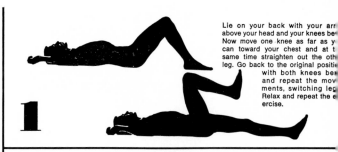

1 Lie on your back with your arms above your head and your knees bent. Now move one knee as far as you can toward your chest and at the same time straighten out the other leg. Go back to the original position with both knees bent and repeat the movements, switching legs. Relax and repeat the exercise.

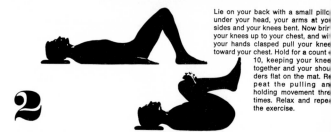

2 Lie on your back with a small pillow under your head, your arms at your sides and your knees bent. Now bring your knees up to your chest, and with your hands clasped pull your knees toward your chest. Hold for a count of 10, keeping your knees together and your shoulders flat on the mat. Repeat the pulling and holding movement three times. Relax and repeat the exercise.

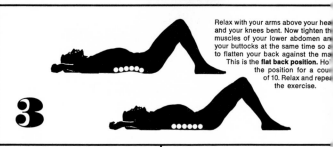

3 Relax with your arms above your head and your knees bent. Now tighten the muscles of your lower abdomen and your buttocks at the same time so as to flatten your back against the mat. This is the **flat back position**. Hold the position for a count of 10. Relax and repeat the exercise.

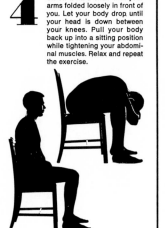

4 Sit on a hard chair with your arms folded loosely in front of you. Let your body drop until your head is down between your knees. Pull your body back up into a sitting position while tightening your abdominal muscles. Relax and repeat the exercise.

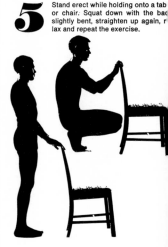

5 Stand erect while holding onto a table or chair. Squat down with the back slightly bent, straighten up again, relax and repeat the exercise.

ow to get along
ith your back

Sitting: Use a hard chair and put your spine up against it; try and keep one or both knees higher than your hips. A small stool is helpful here. For short rest periods, a contour chair offers excellent support.

Standing: Try to stand with your lower back flat. When you work standing up, use a footrest to help relieve swayback. Never lean forward without bending your knees. Ladies take note: shoes with moderate heels strain the back less than those with high spike heels.

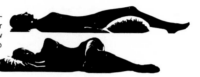

Sleeping: Sleep on a firm mattress; put a bedboard (³/₄″ plywood) under a soft mattress. Do not sleep on your stomach. If you sleep on your back, put a pillow under your knees. If you sleep on your side keep your legs bent at the knees and at the hips.

Driving: Get a hard seat for your automobile and sit close enough to the wheel while driving so that your legs are not fully extended when you work the pedals.

Lifting: Make sure you lift properly. Bend your knees and use your leg muscles to lift. Avoid sudden movements. Try not to lift anything heavy over your head.

Working: Don't overwork yourself. If you can, change from one job to another before you feel fatigued. If you work at a desk all day, get up and move around whenever you get the chance.

Exercise: Get regular exercise (walking, swimming, etc.) once your backache is gone. But start slowly to give your muscles a chance to warm up and loosen before attempting anything strenuous.

our doctor: If your back acts up, see your doctor; don't wait until your condition gets severe.

McNEIL LABORATORIES, INC., Fort Washington, Pennsylvania 19034

FIGURE 14. "EXERCISES FOR LOW BACK PAIN."

(Courtesy of McNeil Laboratories, Fort Washington, Pa.)

following instruction sheets. These are usually accompanied by office demonstrations to clarify any questions regarding any of the exercises.

Shoulder Exercises

1. Pendulum Exercises:
    a. Lean forward and hold on to a table with good hand and hold a 1 to 2 lb. weight, such as canned goods or metal weight, in affected hand; let the arm hand hang loosely with shoulder relaxed. Swing arms forwards and backwards, keeping elbow completely straight, not flexing elbow with motion.
    b. Next swing arm laterally across the body, to the right and left, again keeping elbow straight.
    c. Now begin to make circles, beginning with smaller circles and gradually increasing the size of the circle. Next reverse direction of circles and repeat.
    The arm should swing free like a pendulum during these exercises without using the shoulder muscles. Exercise for approximately 5 minutes, two or three times a day.
2. Raise arms forward and overhead as far as possible, keeping the elbow straight. Try to exceed previous point with each effort.
3. Raise arms laterally away from the sides, bring them overhead and then clap the hands together keeping the elbows straight.
4. Lock hands behind the neck, then pull elbows backwards and throw the chest outwards as the shoulders are extended backwards.
5. a. Place the flat of your hand on your lower back, then gradually try to raise or crawl the hand up the back towards the opposite shoulder. Next repeat with opposite hand, if both shoulders are involved. Try to reach the same point on your back with the affected shoulder as with the normal shoulder.
    b. With hand again held flat across back, grasp a towel thrown over opposite shoulder and held with good hand, grasp with affected hand and pull hand up as far as pain tolerance permits.
6. Wall Climbing:
    a. Stand sidewise to the wall, keeping elbow straight; walk fingers up wall, make a mark, then repeat 10 times and try to exceed the mark each time.
    b. Repeat the same procedure, facing the wall.
7. Take a small stick or baton 2 feet long, lie on back, grasp with both hands and swing hands overhead, using the good arm to force the affected arm backwards. Repeat 10 times.

These exercises should be performed for a total of approximately 15 minutes, repeated 2 to 3 times daily. Exercise until tired but do not exceed fatigue limits. Gradually increase the intensity and duration of exercise period as pain tolerance is increased.

KNEE EXERCISES

1. QUADRICEPS-SETTING EXERCISES:

a. Sit with legs straight on sofa or floor, then tighten kneecap by pulling upward and pressing the back of the knee towards the floor. Repeat this 20 to 25 times. This can also frequently be done while sitting in an automobile with leg outstretched, while waiting for traffic light to change, etc.

b. Tighten quadriceps muscle as in (a), then raise the leg in the straight position 4 to 6 inches off the floor, hold it there 10 seconds, then release. Repeat 10 times.

2. FLEXION EXERCISES:

a. Sit with knee bent or flexed over a table; then straighten knee completely and tighten kneecap; next let leg bend slowly downwards as far as it will go, using gravity and weight of leg. Then, assist flexion of leg by pressing over the ankle of the injured leg with downward pressure of the opposite foot.

b. Lie on stomach and bend leg and knee as far as possible, raising heel towards buttocks; then use your hand to assist and pull the foot as close as possible to the buttocks.

3. PROGRESSIVE RESISTANCE EXERCISES:

Sit with legs flexed over edge of table; use lady's handbag or similar support to hold weights; then raise and straighten knee and leg to the fully extended position with the weight suspended over ankle. Begin with 2 to 5 lbs weight, depending on physical condition and body build; repeat 10 times. Gradually increase the amount of weight and the number of times repeated until 25 lbs can be raised 25 times; progress by alternating an increase in either the weight or the number of repetitions.

After-Cast Care

Instructions for after-cast care are important both for the patient's information and guidance and for the doctor's protection against malpractice suits.

Whenever a cast is applied, adequate instructions should be given to the patient to prevent harmful sequelae and complications. Distribution of a form such as the following, or a small booklet published commercially for this purpose, insures proper instructions for cast management without misunderstanding. It conserves time, answers the usual questions, and provides an excellent defense for alleged failure to properly instruct the patient.

Instructions for After–Cast Care

1. Keep cast dry. Do not get it wet as this will soften the plaster. Use a washcloth around the fingers or toes to avoid wetting the cast.

2. If the fingers or toes become blue or slightly swollen, report this fact immediately to this office. If unable to contact us, go to the nearest hospital emergency room for attention. Swollen or bluish discoloration of the digits indicates the cast is too tight and must be loosened immediately.

3. If there is swelling of the fingers or toes after the initial application of the cast, elevate the extremity to relieve the swelling. When sitting with a leg cast, keep the leg propped up on a stool or hassock for the first few days to allow the circulation to adjust to the additional weight. If there are any questions about the cast, or if there is any apprehension, do not hesitate to call this office promptly.

4. If you have sustained a fracture, it is customary to have pain, but this usually is not excruciating and can be controlled by aspirin or mild narcotics. Should strong narcotics be required, contact this office or go to the nearest hospital emergency room.

5. If an arm cast has been applied, keep the arm in a sling, elevate it at night with two pillows, fingers pointing toward the ceiling.

6. Do not introduce foreign objects into the cast to scratch because it may cause an ulceration of your skin. Watch children closely because frequently they lose coins, toys, etc. down into the cast.

7. Babies should be carefully lifted, always holding the casted leg. If you were advised to remove the baby's cast the night before, soak it in lukewarm water with vinegar (one tablespoon to a quart of water) and peel it off; apply baby oil or lotion to the skin, then report the following day for a new cast. Excessive delay between changes of cast will result in some loss of the correction obtained by the previous casts.

8. Move your toes or fingers as much as the cast permits; active use improves the circulation, stimulates healing, and promotes early return of function after removal of the cast.

9. Patients with an arm cast should exercise the shoulder of the affected extremity regularly and frequently; the casted arm should be raised upward and overhead and out to the side, to avoid stiffness of the shoulder when the cast is removed.

Contrast Baths

Swelling is often a problem after removal of casts from the extremities, especially the foot and ankle. Residual soft tissue thickening and edema often respond favorably to contrast baths which are easily performed at home. Instructions for use of contrast baths should be given in written form, as few patients will remember the exact routine without a printed instruction sheet.

INSTRUCTIONS FOR USE OF CONTRAST BATHS

The purpose of the treatment is to stimulate circulation by a contrast in temperature of the affected extremity. You should use two buckets or two pans of water; if not available, then use a shower spray, sitting on the edge of the bathtub. Always start and end with the hot water. Regular treatments should be taken at least twice daily, three or four times a day if possible—REGULARLY!

TECHNIQUE—4 minutes hot; 1 minute cold; 4 minutes hot; 1 minute cold; 4 minutes hot; 1 minute cold; 4 minutes hot.

Liniment Rubs

Liniment rubs are useful in relieving muscular aches and contusions, and as an analgesic to promote exercise routines for restoration of joint motion. There are many proprietary preparations sold over the counter, most of them with Oil of Wintergreen as the basic ingredient.

The addition of chloroform to methyl salicylate in an olive oil base has been found to be particularly effective and also provides an additional psycho-therapeutic value as it is available by prescription only. The following prescription may be used.

METHYL SALICYLATE	48.0
CHLOROFORM	12.0
OLIVE OIL q.s.	120.0
Misce.	

SIG. USE AS DIRECTED.

INSTRUCTIONS FOR APPLYING CHLOROFORM–METHYL SALICYLATE LINIMENT

1. Apply compresses with towels, wash cloth, or gauze as warm as can be tolerated to the injured or painful area for 15 minutes.
2. Rub liniment into skin area thoroughly for 3 minutes.

3. Apply warm compresses again for another 5 minutes, if it can be tolerated. Do not blister the skin!
4. Repeat process two to three times a day.

Duplicate copies of all prescriptions should be kept and stapled to the records. This is of value for refills and later reference should there be any question of the medication prescribed. Sometimes the patient will state he was never given a prescription, but a carbon copy will refute this claim.

HOSPITALIZATION

The majority of medico-legal patients with musculo-ligamentous injuries, and no fractures, brain or visceral complications, can be treated as office patients with bed rest at home if necessary. The patient should not be hospitalized unnecessarily, as hospital beds are scarce and should be reserved for only those actually requiring such services. Patients may request that they be hospitalized even though they were involved in a relatively minor accident, apparently prompted by the desire to inflate the extent of their injuries and associated disabilities in order to increase their claim for special damages. A few adroit questions may reveal the idea had originated with the plaintiff's attorney. In no instances should the doctor comply unless he honestly believes the patient does require hospital care. The fact that the patient has Blue Cross or similar insurance coverage, so that hospitalization imposes no financial burden, is certainly no reason to hospitalize the patient unless his injuries warrant hospital care.

However, if the patient has genuine injuries with definite objective evidence, then hospitalization for a few days may be indicated to provide proper treatment and permit further observation. Hospital care is usually required immediately after the accident; however, if treatment and observation in the office have failed to produce the desired improvement, the patient may be hospitalized at a later date for further diagnostic studies, such as a myelogram or electromyogram, or for continuous traction to the head and neck or the pelvis and legs. Continuous traction cannot be performed at home, and if this type of treatment is indicated, then hospitalization is advisable. However, when the acute symptoms subside and the patient has improved, he should be promptly discharged.

Physical therapy can usually be given on an outpatient basis; if it is required daily, and the patient lives at some distance from the treating facility, this may be considered an adequate reason for temporary hospitalization, as some of the effects of therapy are dissipated by the long travel to and from the physical therapy office.

Some physicians make a practice of putting patients in the hospital after an automobile accident even though they are not in acute distress. They may hospitalize them for two or three weeks for constant cervical or pelvic traction or other reasons. However, in most instances the patient gets up and goes to the bathroom, removes his traction for meals, does not sleep in traction, etc. Thus he does not have the constant traction for which he was admitted. In effect, the same treatment could be given him as an outpatient, utilizing office and home care. In many instances the purpose of hospitalization is apparently to increase the special damages claim—and also increase the doctor's bill! Neurotic individuals receiving such treatment usually do not respond to it, even in the hospital, because of a failure to recognize their true difficulty. Some doctors put their patients in the hospital two months or more after a minor accident, despite the obvious fact that the maximum need for hospitalization for accidental injuries is immediately after the accident.

Physicians who perform defendant's examinations on a regular basis soon learn to recognize the physicians who treat a great number of plaintiffs and hospitalize a high percentage of their patients, then submit extraordinarily high bills for their treatment. Some even list a charge of fifty dollars for admitting the patient to the hospital—securing a bed—definitely an unethical practice frowned upon by the American Medical Association. More often than not the defendant examination in these cases is completely negative, with no objective findings to substantiate the great amount of treatment previously rendered (often without diminishing the persistent subjective complaints). In many instances the patients are nervous and have obvious emotional problems, which should have been recognized by any trained physician; proper therapy should have been directed toward relief of their mental difficulties, instead of resorting to hospitalization with extensive work-ups for possible organic ailments which never existed.

The physician should be able to recognize emotional and functional problems, and either treat them or refer the patient for consultation, but not put the patient through many unnecessary diagnostic procedures. However, occasionally a complete work-up may be necessary to be sure that no organic lesion is missed; this is justifiable only where there is some objective evidence indicating the need of such examinations. Consultations should be secured when indicated to bolster the doctor's negative opinion if he has been unable to identify any recognizable illness.

Sometimes the treating physician receives diagnostic help from unexpected sources, as exemplified in the following letter from the patient's attorney to his doctor:

> Dear Dr. Brown:
>
> I concur with you relative to your findings of Mr. Robert Scott. In your report, you mentioned his "anxiety overlay" and this client's extreme apprehension as a result of the accident. *It is my feeling that he has developed a traumatic neurosis as a result of this accident.* I have spoken with the family and they are considering having him examined by a psychiatrist in the area, namely Dr. Joseph Anderson. I would appreciate your thoughts in this regard, particularly with the extreme nervousness Mr. Scott has exhibited in my office where he is fidgety, apprehensive, nervous and worried about himself during each and every interview.
>
> Very truly yours,
> E. Phelps Smith, Esq.

This experienced lawyer was very observant, as there were some manifestations of anxiety. He not only made a *diagnosis* but even recommended a medical consultant! However, the patient here described responded promptly to tranquilizers; after an explanation by his treating physician, he himself recognized his nervous problem and did not require psychiatric help. When told of the attorney's letter, he smiled and said, "I think he is just trying to make this a big case,"—an astute observation! The patient continued to work and did not return for any additional treatment.

The doctor should use all available examining procedures to back up his physical findings and recommendations. However, once he has done so, then further unnecessary modalities should be avoided. The patient should be reassured and advised of the negative findings in a direct and forward manner to avoid any misunderstandings; otherwise the patient's feeling of disability increases with every unnecessary diagnostic procedure and with continued ineffective treatment.

There really is no value in continuing physical therapy over many months when no change in the patient's complaints or symptoms has occurred. Overtreatment of injuries to the neck, for example should be discouraged. Functional or emotional problems should be recognized and labeled without delay, and appropriate treatment instituted. Continued treatment designed for an organic type of injury will not prove satisfactory nor achieve any beneficial results in a neurotic patient. Hospitalization two or three months after the accident usually produces no benefit and should be discouraged; it increases the patient's emotional factors, intensifies his belief in his alleged disability, and results in large medical bills which not only hinder settlement but prevent proper treatment by a neuropsychiatrist or reassurance by the family doctor.

The following report of a defendant examination is illustrative:

RE: PENDLETON, NANCY
    11104 Bolling Road
    East Point, Delaware
OCCUPATION: Demonstrator
EMPLOYER: Eastern Gas Light Co.
MARITAL STATUS: Married

SPOUSE: Thomas Pendleton
AGE: 29   Born: 6-30-40, Delaware.

ORTHOPAEDIC CONSULTATION

HISTORY   March 2, 1970
Has been taking Valium®, now reduced to only at night, apparently 5 mg. Patient has been on four or five other types of tranquilizing medications, which caused lethargy and drowsiness, therefore has to be changed. She returned to work about a week ago. Patient regularly works only on week-ends as a demonstrator for Eastern Gas Light Company. She has continued to work since the accident on her weekend employment, although she was in pain.

Patient states that she previously used tranquilizers for other accidents, but she was better before she used a full bottle of medication. Otherwise has been in good health with no other nervous problems. Had surgery to her right knee six years ago for infected scar tissue. Has four children, normal deliveries.

Patient has not been receiving any office treatment since discharge from the hospital two weeks ago. Has a home traction outfit which she uses twice a day for 15 minutes, 15 pounds.

EXAMINATION: Blood pressure 100/70. Pupils equal and react to light and accommodation. Tongue protrudes in the midline. When asked to open her mouth, patient holds her head rigidly and moves her head perhaps 5 degrees, stating that this is what she calls moving, as before she couldn't move it at all. Heart—normal rate and rhythm. Lungs are clear and resonant throughout.

Has 40 pounds grip on the right, 30 pounds on the left, right-handed, Jamar grip tester. Patient states "she's great compared to what she was." In testing sensation patient reports a distinct difference in the left upper extremity, hypesthesia as compared to the right, also involving the left side of her face as compared to the right. In the lower extremities there is less of a difference, although sensation on the left is slightly less distinct than on the right.

Biceps, triceps and radial reflexes are equal and normally active.

In testing cervical motion, patient complains of pain with lateral rotation at 50 degrees, then continues with discomfort to 90 degrees; on the left states she has pain at 70 degrees, cannot go any further, but continues to 90 degrees; 75 degrees forward flexion, 72 degrees extension, complaining of pain with all motions; 45 degrees lateral bending right and left, again complaining of pain while going through these motions.

With patient standing erect with both shoulders abducted to 90 degrees, elbows flexed 90 degrees, she makes a tight fist with the examiner grasping her hands, stating this causes pain to shoot between her shoulder blades and up to her neck, but not to her head. With the patient standing and with examiner grasping her mid-arms, pain shoots from the shoulders up to either side of her neck, but not up to her head, (non-organic manifestations). With fingertip pressure on vertex, patient states she has pain in both ears. She does a good shoulder shrug; has a full range of external and internal rotation, overhead elevation and abduction of both shoulders. With patient standing relaxed, there was no muscle spasm noted in the cervical region. No tenderness in the cervical region, anteriorly or posteriorly. No enlargement of the cervical lymphnodes or thyroid gland. No tenderness or muscle spasm in the lumbar area. Does a good forward flexion and backward extension without difficulty.

X-RAYS: East Point Hospital Center, 1-13-70, *Cervical spine.*
"No evidence of fracture or dislocation. Intervertebral spaces equal and intact. Neural foramina are normal and there are no cervical ribs present."

DIAGNOSIS: No evidence of injury to neck.

PROGNOSIS: It is grossly evident that we are dealing here with an emotional or functional element with gross inconsistency noted throughout the examination and lack of confirmatory objective evidence of the injury. Patient's statements are also grossly inconsistent, stating that this has been a much more serious accident, yet in the other two accidents she was under active treatment for three to five months and had follow-up care for another three or four months, noting that it has been less than four months since this accident. Also, patient states she was *in tears* for six weeks after the accident because of severe pain; yet she worked on week-ends. I fail to comprehend why she received so much treatment and hospitalization three months after the accident when it is so obvious that you are dealing here with a functional nervous element. She is also receiving Valium as a tranquilizer, which would indicate that her doctor has recognized the emotional problem.

In my opinion she requires no further treatment and should be discharged from active care. Patient should also be reassured. She is able to continue with her usual activities.

The alleged hypesthesia of the left side of her body is definitely functional and non-organic in origin, and confirms the above opinion.

Stuart J. Brown, M. D.

The case of Roberta Starr represents prompt recognition of anxiety or functional overlay and early referral for neuropsychiatric consultation and therapy. The probable source of the daughter's nervousness is apparent in the report of the mother's phone call—her home environment undoubtedly contributed to the emotional instability which was exhibited to the doctor after the relatively minor injuries of her auto accident. As so often happens, the family resented the implication and possible stigma of a mental problem and refused to have neuropsychiatric consultation. In this case apparently the mother needed the psychiatric help more than her injured daughter!

RE: STARR, ROBERTA
1919 Allentown Road
Greendale, Virginia

OCCUPATION: Student
MARITAL STATUS: Single
AGE: 15   Born: 9-7-54, Washington, D. C.

ORTHOPEDIC CONSULTATION

EXAMINATION DATE: June 23, 1970
CHIEF COMPLAINT: Injury to right shoulder, neck, hips, 6-18-70.
HISTORY: Patient was a right front seat passenger in a Chevrolet, which had slowed almost to a stop on St Barnabas Road near Back Road, Greendale, Virginia, when struck from the right side by another standard size automobile at 12:30 P.M., 6-18-70. She was taken to West Brook Hospital by ambulance where x-rays were made, given medication and released. She returned on 2 occasions to see the resident physician. Additional x-rays were made but no specific treatment given. She is now complaining of pain in the right shoulder, arm, soreness of the right hip, and pain in the neck. She had fractures of the fingers in 1969 while playing basketball, but has had no other injuries, surgery or serious medical problems.

EXAMINATION: Has 38 lbs grip on the right, 44 lbs on the left, Jamar grip tester, right-handed. Has 75 degrees forward flexion, 60 degrees backward extension; 47 degrees lateral flexion and 90 degrees lateral rotation of the cervical spine. Has pain with the last 10 degrees of lateral rotation of her head and neck to the right. Sensation is intact in both upper extremities. Has some soreness beneath the right rib cage and right breast area, but breath sounds are clear. No friction fremitus.

No rales. Heart—normal rate and rhythm. Lungs are clear and resonant. Pupils are equal and react to light and accommodation. Tongue protrudes in the midline.

Examination of the chest shows some tenderness over the inner end of the right clavicle with swelling here and some prominence.

Patient has definite tenderness and muscle spasm in the right upper trapezius area at the base of the neck posteriorly with pain here with lateral compression and shoulder shrugging on the right. Has some limitation of right shoulder motion.

X-RAYS: West Brook Hospital, 6-19-70, *Left hip:* "Negative. No fracture or dislocation."

West Brook Hospital, 6-21-70, *Both shoulders:* "Normal. Negative for fracture or dislocation."

West Brook Hospital, 6-21-70, *Cervical spine:* "No evidence of fracture or dislocation or subluxation. The study is normal."

This Office, 6-23-70, *Right shoulder:* No evidence of fracture.

DIAGNOSIS: 1. Contusion, right clavicle, moderate.
                      2. Strain, cervical, moderate.

RECOMMENDATION: Patient will receive treatment with hot packs, massage and traction to the cervical area. Also advised to use moist heat and exercises at home. Patient advised to return here for treatment three times a week and will be re-checked after six treatments.

Stuart J. Brown, M. D.

7-2-70

Patient's mother telephoned, stating that the patient's symptoms apparently have become aggravated, with radiating pain to the arm along with a numbness sensation. It is recommended that the patient wear a cervical collar; also placed on Valium, 2 mg tid and Nodular® 150 mg HS. Patient advised to see Dr. Brown in one week.

7-4-70

Patient states she did not understand that she was to get a collar and did not obtain one. Patient states she stayed home the past week because when she is up a couple of hours she feels as if her neck is going to collapse (a good reason to be wearing the prescribed support). Patient has been receiving physical therapy without improvement; the patient reports that she feels worse after receiving the treatments consisting of hot packs, massage and Sayre halter traction.

EXAMINATION: Patient is a fifteen-year-old with an adult-like look and dress, hairdo, etc. Patient demonstrates a full free range of forward flexion, backward extension and lateral rotation, but states it hurts with all these motions except for lateral rotation to the left. There is no tenderness or muscle spasm in the cervical or upper dorsal spine. She bends forward a few degrees and then complains of pain in the mid–dorsal spine. She demonstrates 90 degrees lateral rotation of head and neck to the left without pain, 84 degrees to the right with discomfort at this point. Reflexes and sensation are intact. She has a full range of motion of both shoulders, but patient complains of discomfort and pain with these motions. She states that her right arm swells and feels like it has a fever in it in the morning, and the "whole right hand goes numb when she lays down." She states she has had no response to the Valium (2 mg) and the Nodular.

At this time I do not believe her symptoms are on an organic basis, but probably represent a definite anxiety or functional overlay. Patient will be referred to Dr. George Parker for neurological work-up. Further physical therapy is being suspended until this consultation is obtained.

7-4-70

Mother phoned at 5:40 P.M. and was quite angry, stating that I was not very nice to her daughter (noting that she wasn't even here and knows nothing but hearsay information). She also resented that on the initial visit I told her daughter she was old enough to speak for herself, the mother having intervened and volunteered most of the history. It is my considered opinion that there is a definite overlay here with probable exaggeration of her complaints, possibly due to some parental problem. Under the circumstances, I do not wish to treat this patient any further and am withdrawing from the case. Incidentally, when I came to the phone, the mother hung up in my ear!

Stuart J. Brown, M. D.

SURGERY—SIGNIFICANCE IN MEDICO-LEGAL CASES

When major surgery becomes necessary in a medico-legal case, the entire aspect of the litigation changes and its settlement value is enormously increased. Nothing pleases a plaintiff attorney more than to learn his client requires surgery as a result of the accident in which he represents him! The high costs of hospitalization, the anesthetist's fee, surgical fees, loss of time and wages from work, and the additional pain and suffering all greatly augment his claim for damages, often converting a lower court claim to a Circuit or District Court case.

Performance of surgery of questionable indication and merit greatly complicates a medico-legal case and may make an out-of-court settlement impossible. The situation usually results from chronic complaints from neck and low back injuries which have failed to respond to proper conservative treatment. In almost each incident there is definite evidence of a severe emotional or nervous disorder resulting in continued complaints despite administration of prolonged treatment. In desperation, or in an effort to "get the patient off his back," the doctor sometimes "threatens" the possibility of surgery and then is forced to perform it when the patient agrees. Obviously, surgery is not the answer to an emotional problem, nor does it usually provide a cure. If liability is clear, as in many rear end collisions, the large claim for damages can be sustained even though the operation was not necessary, as the patient followed the recommendations of his or her physician. Cases of this type become almost impossible to settle for a reasonable amount because of the extensive special claims for hospitalization, medical expenses, loss of time from work, among other factors, all resulting from a wrongful indication for surgery.

Sometimes doctors who are interested in a particular surgical procedure will perform a series of such procedures, and are eagerly looking for possible candidates for operation. Recently, there has been a wave of interest in anterior spinal fusion for neck complaints. In certain clinics the procedure is routinely performed in many cases, some with dubious indications or without trial of conservative treatment. If a surgeon of such inclination encounters a medico-legal case in which the financial reward could be considerable, the patient soon becomes another candidate for the series. In some instances the surgery performed has verged upon malpractice, but even this claim could be attributed to the original defendant in an accident case; it was he who started the chain of events leading to the operation.

In one such case a twenty-one year-old girl had a so-called "whiplash injury to the neck" which did not respond to three to four months of conservative treatment. Although she was obviously a very nervous young lady, a suburban physician recommended surgery to relieve her problem and performed an anterior cervical spine fusion, but not in the usual manner. He did not enter the cervical disc space as the patient had no radicular pains; instead he used a Phemister type graft by merely laying a piece of iliac bone along the anterior ligament of the cervical spine, without the usual preparation of a fresh bed of bone. Not only was the patient not relieved of her cervical complaints, but her discomfort became quite real when the graft fractured after removal of the cervical collar. At this time her pain was intense and no longer functional; she was in trouble. The case was settled out of court for forty-five thousand dollars, whereas if the operation had not been performed, the settlement figures had been projected as a maximum from five to seven thousand. The doctor gained not only his surgical fee but also one more case in his experimental series!

In this particular case there was an unusual sequel. Because the defendant's examiner had indicated that there was no logical association of the operation with the minimal injuries sustained in the accident, as well as the unusual nature of the surgery performed in a 21 year-old girl, the plaintiff subsequently filed suit against the orthopaedic surgeon for malpractice. Her attorney sought the help of the orthopaedist who had made the defendant examination, but he declined to become involved. However, medical testimony was secured from other sources and the litigation continued. At this time the result is not known, but it appears that there is a basis for the malpractice suit, and most likely the patient will obtain a substantial recovery. The increasing need for peer review and policing of the medical profession *from within* has been observed frequently for the past several years; cases of this nature demonstrate why our malpractice claims and rates are steadily increasing.

In still another case, a doctor performed a Cloward procedure, removal of the cervical disc and anterior fusion, in a twenty-six year-old female with a history of hysterical breakdown after an auto accident at age fifteen. Despite negative neurological findings by an outstanding neurosurgeon, a negative myelogram, negative electromyelogram, negative x-ray studies of the cervical spine, and no neurological motor or sensory deficit of either arm, the doctor operated. The anterior spine fusion was performed by an orthopaedic surgeon, but in that particular geographic area most of these procedures are performed by neurosurgeons; this implies additional malpractice risk and exposure. The operative description mentioned nothing about instability or the condition of the cervical disc which was removed. The pathology report indicated normal cervical disc tissue with no evidence of degeneration.

One month after surgery the spine fusion was not progressing well by x-ray, but the patient declared she felt fine and had no problems. She felt the operation had cured her of her cervical complaints, although at the one-month stage this was impossible on an anatomical basis. The defendant examiner concluded that this was an unusual approach to the treatment of an emotional problem; her treating physician and a consultant neurosurgeon had previously advocated only symptomatic care. The physician had added another case to the series of anterior spine fusions, for a handsome fee. The defendant examiner was aware that this doctor had performed at least one other such procedure on a medico-legal litigant with like indications and under similar circumstances.

After the surgery the demands for recovery became extremely large. In this case the patient's car was lightly tapped in the rear at an intersection, when her car stalled while taking off from a change of traffic lights; it was struck from behind by a "large fat Cadillac" driven by a well-known builder and public sports figure of substantial means. The case was settled in the middle of the trial after the defendant physician demonstrated the lack of need for such surgery and forthrightly stated that the operation was not indicated under the circumstances; he stated it should not have been performed and was a dramatic overtreatment of an emotional problem. After the trial the defendant attorney spoke with some of the jurors. One stated that he believed the defendant's position that surgery was not required, but he still felt that the patient should have received a substantial sum for her pain and suffering as the operation did result from the accident. Another believed that she deserved absolutely nothing, as he believed all of her symptoms were either feigned or grossly exaggerated (which was true!) This demonstrates the dilemma of an attorney faced with a jury trial—one never knows how jurors react to contrasting medical testimony. Prior to trial the defendant offered twenty-five thousand dollars to the plaintiff, but she demanded a minimum of fifty thousand. The case was settled for thirty thousand dollars during a recess after the defendant physician's testimony that the operation was unnecessary and wrongfully indicated.

Another vivid example of unnecessary surgery in medico-legal cases is illustrated in the following case report, in which prolonged complaints without organic foundation led to radical surgery—lumbar laminectomy and spine fusion. An eighteen year-old girl was involved in a minor automobile accident, followed by initial complaints pertaining to her neck and upper back. She continued to work and did not seek medical attention until two or three days after the accident. Not until six months after the accident did she make any significant complaint about her lower back, although on one occasion she had casually mentioned it to her doctor. No specific treatment had been given to her back, as her principal treatment had been to her neck, and even this was sporadic in nature.

The patient married and immediately became pregnant, following which her back complaints became significant for the first time. At this point the attending orthopaedist noted considerable nervous tension from domestic strife interjected into the patient's increasing somatic complaints. During her pregnancy, the patient became separated from her husband and subsequently divorced him. She had a normal delivery but her back complaints increased. She was given a set of back exercises, various tranquilizer and analgesic medications, and fitted with a back support, and yet none of these gave her relief. She never received a supervised course of physical therapy nor was she hospitalized; she continued to work in a clerical position, without significant loss of time from her job.

Finally, approximately three years after the auto accident, she was admitted to a hospital and a myelogram performed, which revealed only a probable constriction at L-4 and no other abnormalities. Her routine x-rays were reported to show some asymmetry of the facets and minimal narrowing at the L-5-S-1 interspace (this was the interpretation of her attending orthopaedist). No defects were noted in the pars interarticularis, no fractures, no dislocations, no arthritic changes. The patient was otherwise in good health.

Surgery was performed three-and-a-half years after the accident, with exploratory laminectomy at L-4-5 and L-5-S-1 by a neurosurgeon whose findings were entirely negative except for "some instability of the lumbosacral spine"; a routine Hibb's type of spine fusion, L-4 to S-1 was performed by the orthopaedist. The patient had an uneventful post-operative course, and an excellent fusion at L-5-S-1 was noted after two months, followed by a satisfactory fusion at L-4-5. Despite the firm internal stabilization resulting from the fusion, the patient would not discard her brace support and continued to use it periodically, stating that exacerbations of her back pain could only be controlled by the surgical garment. She did admit to having less severe back pain than before surgery, but still claimed she had intermittent episodes of similar pain.

The defendant examiner found excellent fusion at the operative site with only mild restriction of back motion; there were no other objective findings by clinical or x-ray examination. He was unable to logically relate the low back surgery to the accident which had occurred three-and-a-half years prior to her operation. In his report he noted the absence of any back complaints immediately after the accident, also the aggravation of her back complaints by her subsequent pregnancy, and the apparent functional nature of her present complaints. This was demonstrated when the patient complained of pain in the low back with toe flexion and extension in the prone position with her knees flexed 90 degrees, a maneuver in which there is no anatomical relationship. It was also noted by the examiner that had the allegedly unstable lumbosacral spine been really responsible for her back complaints, her complaints should have ceased after the successful fusion and stabilization of the lumbar area. Furthermore, with such a successful fusion, there should be no need for an external back support.

This case was impossible to settle because of the high special damages resulting from her surgery, which the defendant was unwilling to associate with the accident. It was ironical that in this particular case the settlement discussions would probably have been fruitful had the surgery not been performed, as the plaintiff's attorney usually represented defendants and had frequently "crossed swords" with the treating orthopaedist in this case. However, in accordance with the legal obligation to his client, he was forced into litigation because of the radical surgery unnecessarily performed on this patient.

Some patients are surgery-prone and undergo multiple surgical procedures for their continued complaints. Many of their complaints are on a nervous basis which either is not recognized or is given little weight by the treating physician. Surgery produces little change and the patient often has the same complaints or even more difficulty than he had pre-operatively. One such case involved a fifty-one year-old property manager who was initially injured in 1960, in a rear end collision; he had a spine fusion at that time after having a lumbar disc removed in 1950. He also had multiple surgery for bursitis and excision of a torn cartilage in his knee, all within six to seven years prior to the present accident.

Subsequent to the 1960 accident, the patient was involved in another rear end collision in 1961, and then still another rear end accident in 1964. Following the 1964 accident, he had an anterior spine fusion of the neck, and returned to work within two months. He continued to have multiple complaints in his back and neck, then suffered a mild bumper-type accident with almost no property damage, four months after the cervical fusion. Again he continued to complain of vague pains in both arms and hands, numbness, and so on, of his entire left upper extremity and also of the right arm. On examination he was found to be an obviously very nervous individual with a glove type of hypesthesia of the left arm. The patient was quite apprehensive and refused to permit any detailed examination. He complained of pain in his back with toe flexion and extension while lying prone—no anatomical association. X-rays of his neck showed a satisfactory cervical fusion at the C-5-6 level with no adverse effects from the latest accident. The examiner stated that this man needed neuropsychiatric evaluation and possibly treatment.

Two months after the examination by the defendant doctor, the patient was readmitted to the hospital for another spine fusion, this time adding C-6-7 to the previous C-5-6 fusion area. No myelogram or electromyogram was performed prior to the additional surgery. Several months after the additional surgery, the patient was again admitted and a "bone spur" was removed, whereupon he improved. This turned out to be a bone graft plug which had been extruded from the C-6-7 disc space. The patient's pain had been increased by the second operation, but was improved after the extruded plug was removed. Later he continued to a good fusion extending from C-5 to C-7. On examination two years later he had a definite hypesthesia in both arms in a definite functional pattern; he also had hypesthesia of both knees in a circular pattern—three inches above the knee and three inches below the knee joint. His gross nervousness was easily observed.

In review of the case, it was obvious that the patient had been subjected to excessive and repeated surgery with no improvement in his general condition. He had never received psychiatric attention as suggested by the defendant examiner, but instead additional surgical procedures were performed without justification. The case came to trial but was settled during the proceedings because of frank liability and the enormous hospital costs; the patient had the operations whether or not he needed them. This made settlement a very expensive matter as the defendant was legally responsible for the expenses incurred as a result of his accident.

This case graphically illustrates the danger of overemphasizing the patient's subjective complaints and of failing to evaluate a possible psychiatric basis for them, before proceeding with extensive surgical procedures which usually do not improve the patient's condition or relieve his complaints. The motivation of this particular surgeon is difficult to explain, even with generous understanding of the problems that confront the physician in managing a neurotic patient.

REPORTS CONCERNING SURGICAL PROCEDURES

An elective surgical procedure such as arthrotomy of the knee should be carefully considered in litigation cases, as it does complicate the judicial process as noted in the preceding examples. However, if the examiner honestly believes that surgery is necessary to achieve a good result, he should recommend it. In his report he should support his recommendation by stating the basis of his opinion and also give a prognosis for loss of time from work, length of convalescence, and the anticipated result, expressed as degree of residual disability or complete recovery.

Occasionally a zealous plaintiff's attorney will request the doctor to speculate as to what surgery may be required in the future, even though there is no definite indication for operation at that time. This is observed particularly after injuries to the lower back or where there is a possibility of post-traumatic arthritis following a fracture involving a joint. The attorney can then use the report to force a larger settlement, or justify a larger verdict if the case goes to court. When writing such a report at the lawyer's request, the doctor should realize that the case may come to trial, and that he will be subject to cross-examination on that report. If he does not have a firm medical basis to justify his predictions, his entire testimony will be adversely affected. Thus, the doctor should be wary of being trapped into giving information purely for the benefit of the attorney, who states, "Don't worry about it; I'm sure with this statement we will settle the case, you will get your money, and you won't have to go to court." He must remember the defense also has medical witnesses to evaluate the need for surgery and, unless statements are well founded on accepted medical facts, he may be subject to considerable embarrassment and forced to retract his statements, all a result of trying to help an ambitious attorney.

A recent example involved a back injury in which the objective findings by both the treating physician and the defendant examiner were negative, despite the patient's persistent subjective complaints. All of the usual signs of a herniated disc, such as the Lasègue and Naffziger tests, straight leg raising test, reflexes, sensation, muscle power, and x-rays—all were negative. In the opening statement at trial, the plaintiff's attorney alleged permanent disability of the back because of the necessity for surgery, something which had not been mentioned in the pre-trial pleading; this then resulted in a mistrial. Shortly thereafter, the treating physician submitted a long report to the attorney, detailing the prospects of a laminectomy for a possible herniated disc. He then further developed the possibility that the laminectomy might result in instability and this would then lead to a spine fusion. Not content with this amount of surgery, the doctor launched into a discussion of the possibilities of pseudo-arthrosis following the attempted spine fusion, which in turn would result in several attempts at achieving a successful spine fusion. At this point, he did stop in his speculation—one wonders why he did not continue with the possibility of accidental severance of a spinal nerve root leading to paralysis of the lower extremity, post-operative disc space infection, or even death from a post-operative complication such as a pulmonary embolus! His predictions were based purely on the patient's (female) subjective complaints, as when he re-examined her following the mistrial, he again discovered no objective findings, other than a slight limitation of forward flexion of the lower back. No myelogram was performed, nor was one ever proposed prior to the surgical procedures.

From the following letter, it is quite obvious that the doctor was formulating findings for the benefit of the attorney in the next legal proceeding:

The physical findings were entirely negative except for some limitation of forward flexion. There was poor reversal of the normal lordotic curvature of her spine in this maneuver. Straight leg raising tests were negative, and neurological examination of the lower extremities was within normal limits. The previously noted absence of the left knee reflex was not seen at this time. Although the knee reflex on the left was somewhat weaker than on the right, it was definitely present.

A final prognosis cannot, of course, be formulated at this time. I do not feel that there is any question as to the existence of a decompensated intervertebral disc in her lumbar spine. I have spoken at length with Mrs. Rose and it is my impression that conservative therapy would not only be time-consuming, but will not be efficacious in totally eliminating her problem. I have therefore outlined and recommended a course of surgery to Mrs. Rose and she agrees with this course of action.

Generally speaking in removal of a herniated disc, the procedure is obviously of major magnitude, and requires a general anesthetic. For removal of a disc, the usual hospitalization period is seven days, followed by a period of rehabilitation and, during that period of time, avoidance of straining the lumbar region, but at the same time performing exercises designed to strengthen the musculo-ligamentous supporting structures of her spine, in hopes of preventing a recurrence. It is difficult at this time in Mrs. Rose's case to determine whether or not a lumbar fusion will also be necessary at the time of laminectomy. This will probably only be determined at the time of surgery when the joints and other architecture of the lumbar spine will be examined. If a fusion is required, then the hospital stay is usually prolonged and may last anywhere from two to six weeks, assuming no complications occur. Following a fusion, the patient is required to immobilize the area of fusion, which is usually done by means of a plaster of Paris cast, or a fabricated lumbosacral corset. This is worn until the fusion heals, which may take anywhere from four to six months in an adult. Occasionally the fusion does not heal, and this again may require further surgery, and again may prolong the period of hospitalization and rehabilitation.

As concerns the fees involved, the cost of a laminectomy and removal of a disc of course differs with various physicians, but is usually in the range of three hundred to five hundred dollars, whereas if a fusion is performed, depending on the extent of the fusion, this may mean an additional three hundred to six hundred dollars. Generally speaking in hospitals today the cost of a day in the hospital is approximately one hundred dollars, including drugs, operating room fees, anesthetic fees, etc.

Thank you very much. If you have any questions, please do not hesitate to call.

Sidney Davis, M. D.

Many cases are either settled or fail to be settled because of statements written by the attending physician. As previously noted, when surgery is recommended, the entire financial aspect of the case is dramatically altered and it may be difficult to settle if the defendant is skeptical regarding the validity of the recommendation. On the other hand, it may facilitate settlement if the proposed surgery has a firm basis. An experienced defendant examiner is sometimes amazed at the radical surgery proposed in cases he has been asked to evaluate, without substantiating clinical findings; in some instances the fee appears to be the only foundation for the surgical recommendation.

An excellent illustration of this problem is evident in the following case. A twenty-one year-old boy with occasional backache had spine fusion surgery proposed because of minimal sacralization of the 5th lumbar vertebra, congenital type, with no evidence of degenerative changes, spondylolisthesis, or neurological defects. The boy was able to participate in many sports activities and athletics although he did have occasional minimal low back discomfort. The defendant examiner found him to be a rather emotional individual of the so-called "long hair type." An elderly orthopaedist (of good repute, but noted by his confreres for his radical views) who had examined the patient on several occasions, stated that ultimately a spine fusion would have to be done if the boy continued to complain. This medical report resulted in an out-of-court settlement of ten thousand dollars. Before the orthopaedist had made his dour prediction, the case was on the verge of settlement for thirty-five hundred to four thousand dollars, with acknowledged liability, as there were very limited special damages and expenses. However, the insurance company was apprehensive of trial in a rural county courthouse where the only orthopaedist in that community would state that major back surgery would be required; they rightly feared a large jury verdict substantially more than the settlement figure, particularly as there was no question of liability. The defendant's orthopaedist had clearly stated in his report that there was no indication for surgery and substantiated his opinion by detailing the lack of any medical foundation for the proposed surgery. Based on these two contradictory opinions, the plaintiff's attorney settled the case at a lower figure (ten thousand dollars) than had initially been requested (twenty-five thousand to thirty-five thousand dollars) because jury verdicts are upredictable; another factor in the settlement was the defendant orthopaedist's reputation as an expert professional witness.

In another instance involving a woman in her menopausal years, the attending orthopaedist, after having treated the patient conservatively for two years for a traumatic aggravation of a pre-existing osteoarthritis, recommended neck surgery. The patient stated that she had never suffered any previous significant discomfort in her neck. X-ray examination immediately after the rear end collision revealed definite but moderate osteoarthritic spurring with minimal narrowing of C-5-6 and C-6-7 interspaces. Repeated x-rays made at six-month intervals over a two-year period by her attending physician failed to demonstrate any progression of the arthritic changes, and this was clearly stated in the doctor's progress notes. Nevertheless, after two years' time, during which the patient had only moderate symptoms and was able to continue with her housework and other duties, the doctor stated that an anterior spine fusion should be given serious consideration. He prognosticated a very dismal future for this patient as noted in the following letter:

Dear Mr. Sweet:

As I have stated in my most recent report, Mrs. Rachel Best is having moderate difficulty with her neck, documented by limitation of motion and she has had increasing pain over the past several weeks, with the pain radiating up into the occipital area of the head.

The x-ray examination reveals moderate changes at C-5-6 and C-6-7. The patient had these x-ray changes prior to the automobile accident, but there is definitely a causal relationship between the accident of 5-6-68 and the patient's marked difficulty since the time of the accident.

At the present time she is receiving cervical traction. I feel that she will undoubtedly have intermittent difficulty with her neck for the rest of her life and would estimate conservatively the fees in the magnitude of $150 per year for the medical care. If the symptoms remain at the same level then I will recommend an anterior cervical fusion of the involved level. The estimated hospitalization cost and surgical fee with this procedure would be somewhere between $2,500 and $3,000. This procedure is not curative; it simply limits the motion of the involved area and unfortunately there are secondary changes with this limited motion. The usual course of events is that the disc spaces above and below the site of fusion show degenerative changes because of the added strain thrown on these disc spaces and in the period of 4-5 years the patient develops increasing symptoms because of the above described phenomena.

Sincerely,

James Caldwell, M. D.

In his letter the doctor has outlined the cost of hospitalization and surgery, and then discussed the prognosis. It is noteworthy that after surgery he states the patient may have more complaints than previously, because of the resultant limitation of cervical spine motion; he also mentions the possibility of further additional stress placed on the adjacent joints, a valid observation. Nevertheless, he still advocated the procedure despite this poor prognosis of further post-operative discomfort and difficulty.

The defendant attorney, after conference with the orthopaedist who had performed an evaluation on his behalf, concluded that this report had been concocted with doctor-lawyer cooperation in an effort to force a larger settlement before trial. Based on this pre-trial conference he decided to proceed with trial, where he sharply cross-examined the treating physician, pointing out the obvious contradictions of his report. The treating physician retreated in the face of the obvious discrepancies and was forced to admit that perhaps surgery should not be done. The plaintiff's attorney requested a recess at this point, before the next witness (the defendant's orthopaedist) could testify, and the case was settled for the nominal figure of sixty-six hundred dollars; there had been a fifty thousand dollar pre-trial demand.

Another striking example of a medical report addressed to a plaintiff attorney in which the medical consultant overemphasizes the possible complications of surgery is represented in the following case, in which the report includes almost every known post-operative complication, including death. The obvious bias in

this report is evident to any physician, especially if he realizes
that the usual standard for the acceptance of testimony is based
on *probability*, not possibility; there are few (if any) jurisdictions
which permit the entry of "possible" evidence. Most jurors realize
that anything is possible after even the simplest type of surgical
procedure, but they are interested in hearing only probabilities
related to this particular case. When the physician describes each
and every possible complication of surgery and gives a dismal
prognosis, as he does in this case, it becomes obvious that he is
overemphasizing the pessimistic aspects for the financial benefit
of his patient and the referring attorney.

The patient had been involved in two successive accidents,
both involving his neck and back. An orthopaedist examined him
in 1970 on behalf of a defendant for his first accident but at this
time he had also been involved in a second accident (unknown to
the examiner at that time); he re-examined him a year later for
the second accident. Both examinations reviewed the injuries to
his neck and back and both examinations were entirely negative.
The examiner reported numerous functional complaints, such as
alleged pain in the neck when he gripped the patient's fingers,
pain in his back when he moved his toes, etc.

The claimant consulted a prominent neurosurgeon who performed a limited physical examination of his back, reported in six
typewritten lines. His only positive finding was some discomfort
in the back with straight leg raising on the right at 70 degrees.
Many individuals cannot perform straight leg raising past 70
degrees, so that subjective discomfort at this point is not sufficient
to warrant a diagnosis of a herniated disc with a recommendation
for a myelogram and possible laminectomy; a positive straight leg
raising test at a range of 30 to 40 degrees is much more significant.
Despite this lack of an objective basis for his recommendations,
the doctor wrote the following letter to the patient's attorney, re-
markable for the scope of its prognosis:

Re: Louis F. Carson

Dear Mr. Bradley:

Enclosed please find a copy of my letter to Dr. John F. Wallace,
with reference to Louis F. Carson, dated December 28, 1970. As

you can tell from this letter, it was my feeling at that time that the patient probably had evidence of a midline disc with possible protrusion, more on the right than on the left due to the pattern of his straight leg raising. Since I have not seen the patient since that time, I cannot be sure whether the findings remain the same or not. If his findings remain the same, I would continue to recommend hospitalization and possible myelography and/or surgery if he did not respond to a concentrated course of physical therapy. [Note: patient never reported for therapy.]

As you know, any operative procedure has some element of risk. The general experience with lumbar disc surgery is the following: Operative fatalities are quite rare with the incidents usually being reported at approximately 0.4% with most of these being unrelated to the disc surgery itself, but having resulted from emboli or coronary occlusion during the post-operative period. Vascular complications occasionally occur, such as that described in the now famous Jeff Chandler case or cases related to the Samuel Sheppard complications (external iliac tears) for which he recently lost his license in Ohio. Fortunately, the incidence of vascular injury is very, very low. Obviously, any surgical procedure can be associated with a post-operative wound infection, and lumbar disc operations are occasionally followed by infection at the interspace where the surgery was performed. Obviously, injury to the neural elements can also occur. In general, the failure rate of improvement of symptoms after disc surgery amounts to about one in seven to one in fourteen. This is based on recurrence of low back pain with sciatica, and takes into account not only recurrence at the level of surgery, but at any other level in the lumbar area, so that, in general, a person can expect to have an 85% chance of improvement of their symptoms with the risk of their surgery being less than 1% level.

Assuming that he has a good result from surgery, he should be able to return to supervisory work without too much difficulty at the end of one to two months post-operatively; in general, a person after lumbar disc surgery can return to full heavy manual labor, almost any type, within six months.

If I can be of any further help to you, please let me know.

Sincerely,
William Avery, M. D.

It is apparent that the doctor was willing to perform the surgery as he offered the patient a good prognosis for return to work and a realistic outlook for a good result from surgery. The doctor may have been motivated in his listing of possible complications by fear of a malpractice claim for failure of a full disclosure of possible complications. However, the case report reflects poor cooperation by the patient and repeated failure to submit to various plans of recommended treatment. If the doctor's purpose was to protect himself from a malpractice claim, a personal discussion with the patient, after the surgery had definitely been scheduled, would be preferable to a letter to his attorney.

Although this type of report may have some value in negotiation discussions with the insurance carrier, it is doubtful how much weight would be given to it by a jury, especially when the patient did not follow any of this doctor's recommendations.

Undoubtedly the preceding incidents indicate that surgical procedures are sometimes performed with dubious indications and causal relationship to accidents under litigation.

Surgery is often definitely indicated in medico-legal cases, such as to correct deformities, for open reduction of complicated fractures, or for emergency care following serious accidents with resultant major injuries. Immediate operative intervention may be necessary to control bleeding, for abdominal exploration, removal of a ruptured spleen, etc. Open fractures demand immediate surgical care.

In many instances, however, a physical ailment gradually develops or becomes evident over a prolonged period of many weeks or months after an accident, and finally culminates in a corrective surgical procedure. In the following case a partial rupture of the shoulder cuff with tendinitis which was resistant to conservative therapy required surgical correction three months after the bus which the patient was driving was struck by a large tractor-trailer. The patient had a good result and was able to resume his regular occupational duties (Figure 15).

In another auto accident a middle-aged beautician suffered a severely comminuted fracture of the left elbow in which the ends of the humerus protruded through the skin. The patient lay beside her overturned car for eight to ten hours before she was found and brought to a hospital for medical care. Infection developed and retarded healing of the fracture. She developed a

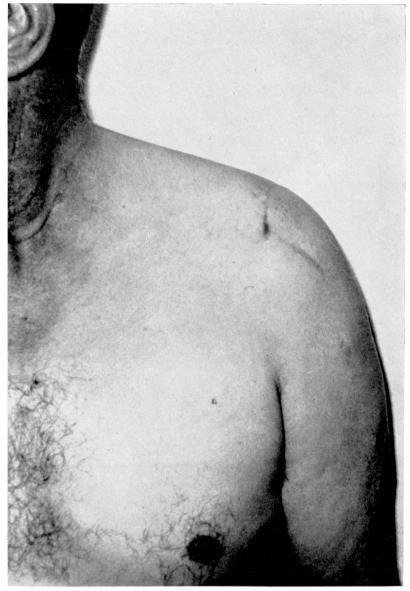

FIGURE 15. SURGERY FOR RUPTURE OF SHOULDER CUFF.
Bus driver with injury to left shoulder. No response to conservative
treatment. Excellent result after surgical repair of partial tear of shoulder
cuff.
A. Surgical scar; minimal atrophy of deltoid muscle.

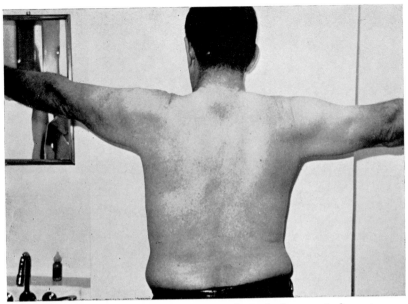

Figure 15. B. Full lateral abduction achieved after surgical repair.

pseudarthrosis which was both painful and disabling. Antibiotics, local wound care, and cast immobilization resulted in control of the infection and cessation of drainage.

Eight months after the wounds had healed a custom-prepared vitallium humeral prosthesis was inserted. The patient tolerated the procedure well and gradually developed a functional range of motion in the left elbow; she extended the elbow to 150 degrees (minus 30 degrees of full extension) and was able to flex the forearm to 75 degrees, or a range of 75 degrees. Pronation and supination were moderately restricted but the patient was able to bring her left hand to her mouth and use it to a limited extent in her work as a beautician. However she also had a partial paralysis of the radial nerve which impaired her hand and wrist function and added to her elbow disability.

The pre-operative pseudarthrosis of the left elbow is demonstrated in the accompanying x-rays. The vitallium prosthetic replacement is illustrated as it appeared six months after surgery, then three years later. She has had no further complications and is satisfied with the results of the elbow arthroplasty (Figure 16).

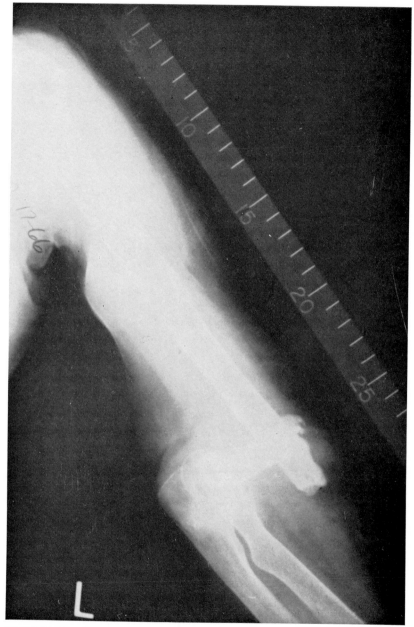

FIGURE 16. SURGICAL CORRECTION OF NON-UNION OF FRAC-
TURE OF ELBOW WITH VITALLIUM PROSTHESIS.
  A. Severely comminuted fracture, with non-union, lower end of humerus,
     eight months after injury.

PROGNOSIS

The prognosis should include a summary and evaluation of the injuries and medical conditions related to the accident (some examiners place this under a heading entitled "Discussion"). A

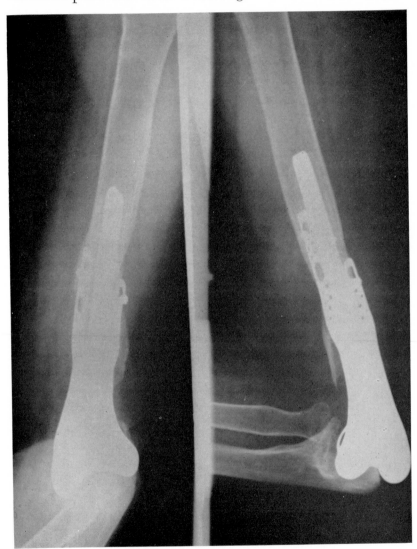

Figure 16. B. Left elbow: Vitallium prosthetic replacement for lower humerus; six months post-operative.

review of any previous medical reports, hospital records, laboratory and x-ray reports, or treatment may be inserted at this
point. If indicated the examiner may discuss causal connection
of pre-existing conditions and traumatic aggravation, such as

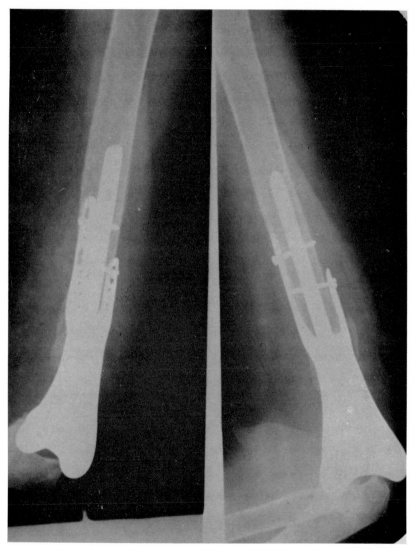

Figure 16 C. Three and a half years after surgery.

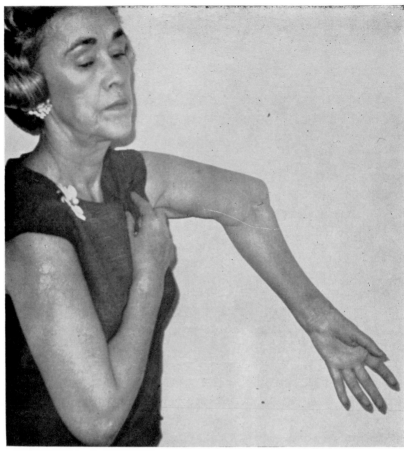

Figure 16 D.

arthritis, postural defects, deformities, and so on. The discussion should be limited to an objective appraisal of the patient's condition, avoiding subjective impressions whenever possible, although the subjective impressions of an experienced examiner are often of value. The question of exaggeration or even possible malingering should be mentioned if pertinent, especially if the objective findings do not substantiate the patient's varied and consistent complaints, and the anxiety factor is minimal. It is usually wise to avoid a definitive declaration that the patient is a malingerer; but the possibility can certainly be mentioned.

If the patient is under treatment, the examiner may anticipate the amount and type of additional treatment required, and
also evaluate the benefit received from previous treatments. Comment may also be included regarding further need of a brace
or support.

If the patient is still out of work, the doctor should state
the date of anticipated return, recording the type of work the
patient had been performing and what is now feasible for him;
this is of value to an attorney who must estimate damages. Often
an early return to work may alleviate a nervous or functional
overlay and divert the patient's attention away from his medical
problems; functional problems are often diminished or eliminated
by occupational activity.

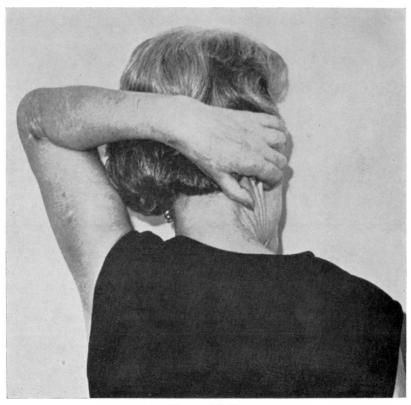

Figure 16 E.

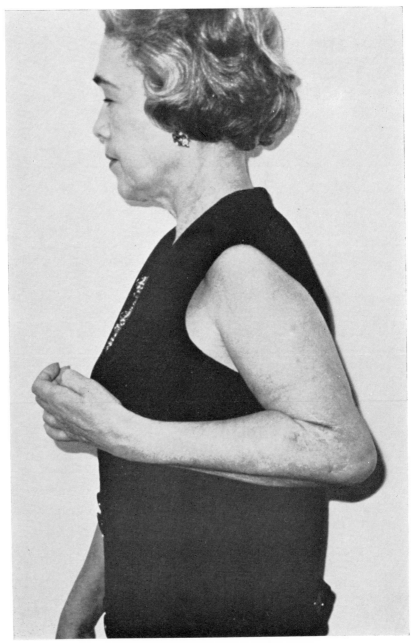

Figure 16 F. D, E, and F: Residual deformity but satisfactory range of motion for useful function.

In Workmen's Compensation cases the examiner should make a definite statement to indicate the anticipated date of return to work, as this is essential for continued payments for loss of time. Sometimes the history and findings indicate the patient should obviously have returned to work long before, but it is difficult for the doctor to make such a statement if he has not examined the patient before and is not personally familiar with his previous condition.

Under Workmen's Compensation law the final physical evaluation and report must include a statement regarding the presence and extent of residual disability. The *American Medical Association Guide for Permanent Impairment* and the recent *Manual of the American Academy of Orthopaedic Surgeons* may be utilized in making an estimate of disability; however, the figures given in these guides do not necessarily apply to any given case, and certainly cannot reflect the examiner's personal opinion. No one is in a better position than the examiner to make an evaluation of a particular case, as he has medical, functional, social, economic, and objective components available to him in addition to the established tables of impairment found in the approved publications. The examiner should familiarize himself with the basic rules of disability evaluation for Workmen's Compensation cases, noting for example that disabilities of the lower extremities are stated in percentages of either the foot or the whole lower extremity, never in terms of the leg or knee.

The physician must exercise care not to develop a stereotyped report which is obviously partisan; the report should neither embellish nor belittle the claim. The physician who acts as an advocate soon receives a label of "insurance doctor" or "plaintiff's physician," which greatly diminishes the value of his reports and testimony, as this reputation becomes apparent to judges, insurance adjusters, attorneys, and hearing examiners. Judges who try numerous accident cases are keenly perceptive of the professional integrity and credibility of physicians who are frequently involved in medico-legal cases. A partisan reputation is gained by the defendant examiner who "never finds anything wrong with the plaintiff," or the treating physician who always gives a pessimistic prognosis amplified by a recital of remotely possible sequelae and disability. On the other hand the report of a competent, unbiased examiner with an established reputation is often mutually acceptable to both parties; if he is the treating physician, frequently the defendant insurance company will not request an independent evaluation of the injuries. If such a reputation can be justifiably earned, the physician can be sure he has not only been practicing good medicine but has also been fair and accurate in his medico-legal appraisals (Figure 17).

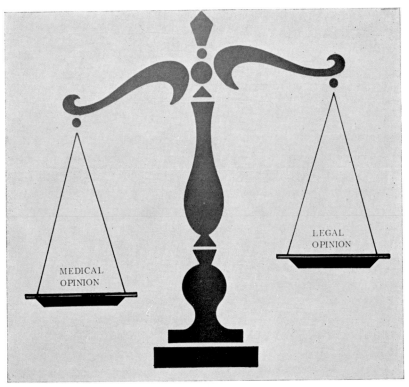

FIGURE 17. AN IMPARTIAL MEDICAL OPINION CARRIES WEIGHT.

4 MEDICAL REPORTS

THE PREPARATION OF MEDICO-LEGAL REPORTS WHICH SHOW COMPETENCE, LACK OF BIAS AND OFFER CONCRETE, PROFESSIONAL ADVICE, IS SOMETHING THAT IS NOT ALWAYS EASY FOR THE PHYSICIAN. OUR PURPOSE HERE IS TO SUGGEST TYPES OF REPORT, FORMATS, ORGANIZATION, DOCUMENTATION, REFERENCE TO HOSPITAL RECORDS, PRESENTATION OF FINDINGS, ETC. THAT SHOULD FACILITATE THIS TASK.

FORMAT

The examining or treating physician should adopt a standard format for his medical reports, with headings and subheadings. This will facilitate preparation of the reports by his secretary and make them more comprehensible to the claims adjuster or attorney who reads them. Here are some suggested titles:

(1) CHIEF COMPLAINT   (5) X-RAYS
(2) PRESENT ILLNESS   (6) DIAGNOSIS
(3) PAST MEDICAL HISTORY   (7) PROGNOSIS
(4) PHYSICAL EXAMINATION   (8) DISCUSSION

Enough carbon copies should be supplied for distribution to all involved parties, usually a minimum of three copies plus a file copy.

At the top of the first page there should be information essential for identification of the patient, such as name, address, age, place and date of birth (helpful in identifying patients with similar names), name of spouse (and address if different), social status, occupation, and place of employment. If the patient was referred by another physician, this can be inserted just before the first heading; no mention should be made in the report of the

171

patient's being referred by an attorney or insurance company. If the examination is for the defendant, the case should be identified by case number if known and the name of the insured, i.e. "vs Joseph Green."

Reports should be dictated or written promptly. As explained earlier, data may be dictated by the physician as the examination proceeds or soon thereafter; the report can then be completed, out of the presence of the patient, by adding the diagnosis and conclusions. With the adoption of a standard operational procedure of this type, it should be possible to forward a report within two or three days after an examination. Prompt submission of a medico-legal report facilitates disposition of the claim and continuation of Workmen's Compensation payments to a disabled employee. Considerable litigation has been settled out of court as the result of a thorough, objective examination and a well-written precise medical report, received before the trial date. Unfortunately, some physicians delay forwarding their reports for so long after the examination (sometimes as long as two to three months) that the value and significance of the report are greatly diminished, whether for the patient or the defendant party. In many instances a possible settlement out of court is lost because of the long delay. Physicians who encounter medico-legal problems infrequently and are not prepared to formulate their reports quickly, may substitute a temporary telephone report to the interested party to facilitate legal procedures, and submit a formal report at a later date.

Medical records forwarded to the physician for preliminary review to aid in his evaluation of the plaintiff should be returned with his report, unless he has been advised to retain them for possible use at trial.

The importance of the doctor's medical reports in the disposal of personal injury cases was stressed by Judge Stevens Fargo of the Los Angeles Superior Court in an address made to the National Medicolegal Symposium in March 1965. He urged that the medical profession give greater attention to the preparation of medico-legal records, noting that a great percentage of personal injury claims are disposed of on the basis of fair and complete reports without a court appearance by the physician. The importance of great care on the part of the physician in preparing his records was observed, since he may be confronted with his own written language in a court appearance. He stressed the need for pre-trial conferences, particularly for the doctor inexperienced in courtroom appearances: "The doctor who feels he does not require any assistance from a lawyer is headed for serious trouble in the courtroom."[8,28]

A. Plaintiff Reports

The following is a typical example of a report after examination of a plaintiff injured in a recent automobile accident. The history recites the importance of medical facts regarding the palintiff's injury and subsequent treatment. It does not delve into the legal issues but confines itself to the medical problems. The examination is reported in detail with emphasis on objective observations and measurements, utilizing available scientific devices. A specific program of treatment is recommended, but no definite prognosis is offered. The physician should be wary of making any statement after the initial examination, which may later prove erroneous and cause subsequent embarrassment.

TYPICAL PLAINTIFF EXAMINATION REPORT

RE: SMITH, EDNA
    105 Upper Branch Road, N. W.
    Washington, D. C.

AGE: 38   Born 1-2-26, Upper Marlboro, Maryland.
DATE: October 15, 1964
OCCUPATION: Housewife
MARITAL STATUS: Married
HUSBAND: John W. Smith
REF: Lester Jones, M.D.

ORTHOPAEDIC CONSULTATION

EXAMINATION DATE: October 14, 1964

CHIEF COMPLAINT: Injury to head and neck, 10-13-64.

HISTORY: Patient states that the Vokswagen sedan which she was driving on Connecticut Avenue, N. W., at about 12 noon, 10-13-64, was stopped for a traffic light near Albemarle Street, N. W., when it was struck in the rear by another automobile, which in turn had been propelled into her car after being struck in the rear by a truck. Patient was stunned and "shook-up," but was not unconscious. She was able to get out of the car but noticed immediate discomfort in her head and neck, then became very nervous. She took a taxi from the scene of the accident and went to the office of her family physician, Dr. Lester Jones, who examined her, gave her a sedative, and then referred her to this office for orthopaedic consultation.

Patient is now complaining of a violent headache, pain at the base of her neck, stiffness of her neck, and difficulty in moving her head from side to side. She had great difficulty in sleeping last night. Also complains of some discomfort in her upper back when she reaches upwards with her arms.

Patient at first stated she had never had any previous similar difficulty with her head, neck or shoulders. However, our records indicated that she was treated in this office on 5-10-56 after a similar type accident with strain of the dorsolumbar area of the mid back and neck from which she recovered after one month of treatment. (Patient recalled this after her nervousness subsided.)

PAST HISTORY: Patient has otherwise been in good health. She had surgery for an ovarian cyst 10 years ago. Laceration of left leg was sutured 5 years ago. No other injuries or serious medical illnesses. No history of treatment for nervousness, hypertension, ulcers, etc.

EXAMINATION: Patient is in obvious acute distress, nervous, and apprehensive, supporting her head with her hands. Blood pressure 122/88. The heart was normal in rate and rhythm, with no murmurs. Her lungs were clear and resonant with full, symmetrical chest expansion. No tenderness or friction fremitus about the rib cage. There is no evidence of injury to her ears, eyes, nose, mouth or throat with no bleeding from these areas; tongue protrudes in the midline; no nystagmus; no facial weakness. Pupils equal and react to light and accommodation.

Satisfactory grip with 33 lbs grip on the right, 26 lbs on the left, right-handed, tested with Jamar dynamometer. Biceps, triceps and radial reflexes equal and normally active in both upper extremities. Sensation, including pin prick, light touch and vibration sense, normal in both upper extremities. Radial pulse equal in both wrists; skin temperature and color symmetrical and normal.

Shoulders are symmetrical and level, with no deformities of the acromioclavicular joints. No tenderness, no muscle spasm, no swelling about the shoulder cuffs. Has full overhead elevation of both shoulders, but with some discomfort at the base of the neck. Has no weakness of the biceps, triceps or deltoid muscles against resistance. Shrugging of the shoulders using the upper trapezius muscles causes discomfort, especially against resistance.

Cervical spine motion is limited, as tested with the Cervigon apparatus; 45 degree lateral rotation to the right, 48 degree lateral cervical rotation to the left, with pain with both of these motions; 65 degree forward flexion and 35 degree backward extension, with further extension limited by pain and muscle spasm; 32 degree right lateral flexion, 30 degree left lateral flexion, further motions again limited by pain and muscle spasm. Lateral cervical compression test causes discomfort at the base of the neck with testing on either side, but no radiation of pain to either upper extremity. Definite tenderness and muscle spasm localized in the upper trapezius area bilaterally, in the suprascapular region, right and left. Lateral arm traction causes no significant pain in the neck. No definite tenderness over the brachial plexus with palpation in the lateral cervical areas.

Good range of motion in the lumbar area, with no tenderness or muscle spasm, and no restriction of low back motion.

X-RAYS: THIS OFFICE, 10-14-64, *Cervical spine* (with oblique, flexion, extension views): No fracture or dislocation. Intervertebral spaces equal and intact. No cervical ribs. Neural foramina are intact and clear. No arthritic changes noted. Restricted range of flexion and extension motion. Some straightening of the normal lordotic curve.

DIAGNOSIS: Strain, moderately severe, cervical spine.

PROGNOSIS: The findings indicate the above diagnosis as a result of the accident of 10-13-64, but the symptoms are enhanced by a definite anxiety overlay associated with this accident. Treatment commenced with physical therapy, including hot packs, and massage to the neck, followed by progressively increased Sayre halter traction, using the tractolator intermittent traction apparatus. She was advised to rest at home and use warm showers or moist heat; a gradually increased exercise program will be added when the acute symptoms subside.

She was given Equagesic® medication as a tranquilizer and muscle relaxant. A cervical collar may be added for temporary support if her acute symptoms persist; also advised to sleep with a small pillow on a firm mattress; to refrain from housework activities until her condition improves.

Patient will return for further treatment three times a week for the first two weeks, then return for further treatment as indicated by a check-up examination. Exact prognosis cannot be given at this early date, until her response to treatment has been evaluated, but patient was reassured that she should continue to a satisfactory result.

Everett J. Gordon, M. D.

B. Defendant Reports

Defendant reports vary considerably depending on the time elapsed between the accident and the defendant exam, amount of treatment, intensity of the patient's complaints, emotional and psychological make-up of the patient, type of treatment, and many other factors.

Most plaintiffs will report subjective complaints to the defendant examiner, even though they have long since been discharged by their treating physician and have resumed normal activities. Some of these may be valid but in many instances the patient is trying to impress the examiner in order to secure a more favorable report. Occasionally, however, a plaintiff will report no residual complaints or impairment; almost all of these individuals are negotiating directly with an insurance adjuster and have no attorney representation.

The following two examples illustrate contrasting patterns of defendant examinations:

1. *(Norman W. Harris)* This report represents a case with minimal injuries, but which resulted in loss of three months' time from work. The patient had only a moderate amount of treatment and had minimal residual complaints for which a defendant examination was conducted within four months after injury. The defendant examiner found no objective residuals of injury, but did find some evidence of exaggeration (Gordon toe flexion-extension test). This type of case is usually settled without necessity for litigation after distribution of an objective defendant report.

2. *(Harriet T. Kramer)* This report reflects a more difficult and complicated defendant examination, requiring evaluation of the need and result of major spine surgery. The patient had prolonged symptoms for several years, based on an apparent large

functional overlay. The indications for surgery were questionable and could not logically be related to the automobile accident under litigation when viewed impartially. However, the treating physician stated there was a causal relationship between the accident, her persistent back problem, and the corrective surgery; the last was only partially successful in relieving her subjective complaints despite an excellent operative result. The affirmative opinions of the surgeon and the subsequent surgery vastly increased the special damages and plaintiff's demand, prohibiting an out-of-court settlement.

Extensive medical records were forwarded for review but were received after the examination had been completed (but before the report was forwarded). The records would have had more value had they been received before the examination. A review and written abstract of these records should be made and forwarded with the examiner's report. The records are not only helpful to the defendant's physician in preparing for the examination, but the abstracted report also aids the layman insurance adjuster or attorney by emphasizing the important facts.

This type of examination requires more time and study than the previous case and merits a higher fee.

1. TYPICAL DEFENDANT EXAMINATION REPORT

August 18, 1971

RE: HARRIS, NORMAN W.
    2601 Jefferson Lane
    Washington, D. C.

AGE: 36   Born: 7-16-35, New Jersey.
EMPLOYER: Independent Tours
OCCUPATION: Bus driver
MARITAL STATUS: Married
SPOUSE: Eve

ORTHOPAEDIC CONSULTATION

EXAMINATION DATE: August 17, 1971

CHIEF COMPLAINT: Injury to left arm, elbow, lower back, 4-16-71.

HISTORY:	Patient was a right front seat passenger, belted, in a compact car which was struck on the left side at 14th and P Sts., N. W. on 4-16-71, about 5:00 P.M. Patient states his car was stopped to enter a parking lot when it was struck, and it was turned completely around. Patient did not go to work that day, but the next evening saw Dr. Davis, who kept him under treatment until the end of June. Patient states he got a needle in his back every time he went to Dr. Davis, 3 times a week, exact number of shots not known. Stayed under his care for a couple of months. Returned to work about a month ago as a truck driver, same as before, and is now working regularly.

Patient states that he still has a little soreness in his back after getting up in the morning or after driving around in his truck all day. Points across the mid lumbar region as the site of discomfort. Has no further trouble with his left arm or elbow.

Never had any previous similar difficulty. Has actually always been in good health. Never had any other serious illnesses, injuries or operations.

EXAMINATION:	Patient sits comfortably in no acute distress. Blood pressure 140/90. Heart—normal rate and rhythm. Lungs are clear and resonant. Patient has a moderately heavy build with a fairly large protuberant abdomen, mild lumbar lordosis. Pupils equal and react to light and accommodation. No discharges, no weakness.

Stands erect with pelvis and shoulders level. Bends forward, fingertips easily touching the floor. Good range of lateral flexion and backward extension without discomfort or restriction. With forward flexion, there is rounding and reversal of the lumbar curve, indicating lack of any muscle spasm in this area. Increased sensitivity over the gluteal portion of the sciatic nerve. No tenderness about the trochanteric regions of the hips. Full range of motion in both hips, including abduction, adduction, flexion and extension, internal and external rotation. Full flexion and extension of the knees with good muscle power without pain or restriction. Leg length 34¼ inches on the right and left. Calves and thighs are symmetrical, measured at comparative distances from medial malleoli. Knee jerks and ankle jerks are equal and normally active. Sensation, including pin prick and vibration sense are intact in both lower extremities. The skin temperature and color are symmetrical. No swelling of the ankles. Has good power of toe flexion and extension, with no weakness demonstrated. Able to walk on toes and heels well. Straight leg raising accomplished to 90 degrees without pain or other difficulty. Lasègue, Naffziger and Patrick tests are negative bilaterally. Patient is able to turn over on the examining table without any obvious difficulty.

With patient lying face down in the prone position, knees flexed 90 degrees, patient complains of definite discomfort and pain in the mid lumbar area as a result of toe flexion and extension (no anatomical association between maneuver performed and alleged increased discomfort).

Patient hyperextends the mid back and upper back well without difficulty. There was no tenderness to palpation in the lumbar area after the alleged pain with toe flexion and extension, which has no anatomical basis. Good range of motion in both shoulders, both arms, with no evidence of injury or loss of function here.

X-RAYS: THIS OFFICE, 7-6-71, *Lumbosacral spine, pelvis and hips:* intervertebral spaces are equal and intact. No fracture or dislocation. Joint spaces are clear. No arthritic changes. Mild increase in lumbar lordosis.

DIAGNOSIS: No evidence of residuals of injury to the left arm, lower back or left elbow.

PROGNOSIS: At this time there is no evidence of residuals of injury by clinical or x-ray examination. Patient's complaints of pain in the lower back with toe flexion and extension represent a definite exaggeration with no anatomical basis for this complaint. In my opinion he requires no further treatment and is able to continue working at his regular job.

Everett J. Gordon, M.D.

2. Typical Defendant Examination Report

August 25, 1971

RE: KRAMER, HARRIET T.
   1974 Windham Ave., Apt. 290
   Arlington, Virginia

AGE: 23   Born: 3-4-48, Mississippi.
OCCUPATION: Librarian
EMPLOYER: Bureau of the Census
MARITAL STATUS: Divorced
VS: Mary Ellen Kane

Orthopaedic Consultation

EXAMINATION DATE: August 24, 1971

CHIEF COMPLAINT: Injury to low back, 4 to 5 years ago (exact date not recalled).

HISTORY: Patient was involved in an automobile accident when she was a passenger in a Chevrolet about 4-5 years ago (exact date not recalled), accident occurring at 33rd and N St. N. W., when their car was hit from the rear by another similar size car. Patient states she never had any previous back problems. Patient promptly consulted Dr. Samuel Abbott, who had previously treated her for a foot problem. X-rays were made and she was given a back brace which she wore for six months. Patient states she had no pain the day of the accident, but the next day she went to work and had such severe low back pain she could hardly stand. She met Dr. Abbott the following morning at Morningside Hospital Emergency Room. She was given the brace and exercises. No other physical therapy.

Patient was off work for a couple of weeks from her summer job, then returned to school in the fall. She became pregnant in 1968, had a normal delivery, 4-29-69, but had phlebitis and periodic low back pain throughout the pregnancy. Patient states that previously she felt her back become tired and she had to wear a brace periodically and avoid the physical education classes in school. Had intermittent discomfort after the pregnancy, during which she wore her brace periodically.

She visited Dr. Abbott approximately 3 times prior to her surgery on 3-12-70 at Morningside Hospital, at which time a lumbar spine fusion was performed. She had a myelogram performed just prior to the operation by a neurosurgeon, Dr. Jack Balance, who participated in the surgery. Patient previously had fallen up steps, after her pregnancy, which Dr. Balance told her was due to a dropped foot. Patient states she began falling about a month and a half before the surgery; not sure which foot, but believes both feet were weak. Pain did continue down both legs and both feet were numb.

She wore a steel brace post-operatively for 4 to 5 months. Patient states she still uses the brace while carrying her baby or doing house cleaning, otherwise has severe pain for several weeks (unusual after a successful spine fusion). Patient states she generally feels much improved, previously had constant pain, now intermittent. She still has dull pain and tingling in her feet, particularly at night when she goes to sleep. Never had any sharp radiating pains from her back down her legs. Tingling in her feet is similar to that pre-operatively, but noted now only if she doesn't wear her brace when she does hard work.

She had no previous back problem. Patient states she had stomach ulcers which she feels have been present since high school. She takes Maalox® or Belbarb® prn. Took 3 Maalox this morning as her ulcers were bothering her today (probably anticipating this exam). Never had any nervous problems. Has not used tranquilizers. Patient states she has had hypermobile joints since she was born, with occasional sprain and muscle tears. Patient was out of work for 2 months after surgery, but is now working regularly as a librarian.

EXAMINATION: Patient has hyperextension of both elbows with 20 degrees of hyperextension in both elbows. Also hyperextends the MP joints of both hands, typical of a congenital hyperelasticity of the joints. Blood pressure 112/74. Weight is 140 lbs, height 67½ inches.

There is a well healed mid line scar, 4½ inches long in the lumbosacral area, not adherent. No keloid formation, not sensitive. Plumb bob falls in the mid buttock crease; there is a right upper dorsal left lumbar curve, compensated. Pelvis level. She bends forward fingertips 5½ inches from floor with no demonstrable motion in the lumbosacral area. There is rounding of the upper lumbar region. She has a good range of lateral flexion, lateral torsion and backward extension with no demonstrable motion at the fusion site and no muscle spasm. No discomfort with these motions.

Leg length is equal, 35 inches bilaterally. Calves are 13⅞ inches in circumference measured 11 inches above medial malleolus. Thighs measured 23 inches above medial malleoli are 18 inches right, 17½ inches left. Straight leg raising easily accomplished to 90 degrees. Full range of motion in hips and knees. Sensation, including vibration sense, pin prick, and light touch, equal and normally active in both lower extremities and feet. Full toe flexion and extension without difficulty. Knee jerks and ankle jerks equal and normally active. Hyperextends the mid back and upper back well against gravity and holds it well against resistance; accomplished without pain, or demonstrable motion in the lumbosacral area. Hyperextends both hips well without difficulty. Walks without a limp. She gets up and down from the examining table with alacrity and without any pain or discomfort. Patient did not bring the brace to the office with her, or use it in driving here.

X-RAYS: THIS OFFICE, 8-24-71, *Lumbosacral spine, pelvis, both hips* with oblique and lateral flexion-extension views: The facets at L-4-5, L-5-S-1 are obliterated and fused. There is no demonstrable motion at the L-4-5, L-5-S-1 level. The remainder of the lumbosacral spine is normal. Evidence of laminectomy performed at right L-4-5, L-5-S-1.

DIAGNOSIS: Post-operative spine fusion, L-4-S-1.

PROGNOSIS: Patient has a generalized increased elasticity of her ligaments, which is a congenital condition. Actually this type of individual is less subject to strain than one with the usual fixed, firm ligamentous structures. In reviewing the history it is noted that patient had no pain the day of the accident, which would not be true if she had a severe injury. In addition, she had very little treatment, no physical therapy and missed very little time from work or other activities, again an indication of a minimal type of injury.

I cannot explain the "falling up stairs" complaints, unless it were due to a drop foot, but she complains bilaterally, which is not generally true with a herniated disc. The records indicate that she did not have a herniated disc at surgery; there is no definite explanation given for her alleged difficulty in falling up stairs and weakness of her lower extremities.

At this time she has an excellent result from the spine fusion with no demonstrable motion in the lumbosacral area and no positive objective findings by clinical examination. With such a good result I cannot comprehend the need of a brace as she already has fixed internal bracing from the fusion; a brace is not required after a successful spine fusion. It is quite possible that this has become a fixed idea with her and it may well represent a strong functional overlay.

The indication for the operation is difficult to comprehend unless it be on a congenital basis. I cannot logically associate it with the accident of 4-5 years ago as had the accident caused sufficient disability and pain, surgery would have been required at a much earlier date and there would have been a greater degree of disability and a greater need for treatment immediately following the accident. It appears likely that her recent pregnancy may have aggravated her back condition and this in itself could have precipitated the need for surgery.

Patient still has vague complaints at present, such as tingling of her feet at night, which I cannot associate with any organic pathology. At this time she appears to have made a good recovery from surgery and requires no further treatment; she does not require the use of a back brace, which she was not wearing at this visit.

Everett J. Gordon, M.D.

August 25, 1971
Re: Harriet T. Kramer
Vs: Mary Ellen Kane

REVIEW OF RECORDS

Dr. Abbott's report of 8-28-67, indicates that the patient was seen because of tightness of her neck in an accident of 8-20-67. Examination of 8-22-67 showed she had mild tenderness in the posterior cervical and mid dorsal area. X-rays were made of the cervical region only. Given a soft collar and extended lumbosacral support. There is not a word in his report about injury to the lumbosacral area or complaints to justify the support for the lumbosacral spine. Examination of 8-28-67

showed some tightness in her neck, no mention of low back examination or findings.
12-22-67

States that her neck and back are moving freely. Only problem was fatigue. Given Williams' exercises.
1-14-69

Patient was pregnant with some back pain. Noticed a lot of tension regarding her marriage. Some tenderness in low back. Dr. Abbott felt she was having some aggravation by her pregnancy and a domestic problem. Advised maternity back support.
11-20-69

Doctor noted low back pain in spite of the use of brace and exercises. X-rays at that time showed some early narrowing at L-4-5, which he felt was different from the x-rays made in August 1967. (No mention made in report of August 1967 of x-rays of the lumbosacral spine). He noted some asymmetry of the facets, which he feels was aggravated by the accident. No surgery recommended.
2-17-70

He noted some absent reflexes, L-4-5 distribution. Also noted loss of sensory pattern. Deferred myelogram.
5-19-70

Patient was doing well. Brace was adjusted.
8-26-70

She was going without her brace. X-rays showed good stability of L-5-S-1. (Apparently patient had had her surgery performed.)

On 1-28-71, she had good stability at L-5, some motion at L-4.

OPERATIVE RECORDS, 3-12-70: Dr. Abbott reports that laminectomy by Dr. Balance found no disc pathology L-4-L-5. He found marked instability and performed fusion from L-4 to S-1. A myelogram on 3-10-70 showed possible constriction at L-4.

The hospital records indicate a final diagnosis of unstable lumbar spine. Dr. Abbott's admitting note states that patient was having persistent pain in her legs and that she had not done well with conservative treatment. He felt that she may have had a disc at L-4-5 from his interpretation of the myelogram that was performed.

Dr. Balance's operative note reports a normal intervertebral disc at L-4-5 and L-5-S-1 interspaces. He explored on the right side L-4-5 and L-5-S-1.

The post—operative note shows that patient did well without complications, and was afebrile.

IMPRESSION: After review of these records (which were received after I had performed my examination and written my report) I have no change from my initial impression and report. I cannot find any definite reason for the surgery performed. In my opinion the reports do not indicate sufficient pathology that would warrant as radical procedure as a spine fusion. It is noted that she had no significant low back complaints immediately after the accident, which would certainly not be true had she suffered any significant injury in this accident of 1967. I believe that there was a great deal of anxiety element present; the patient informed me that she had separated from her husband during her pregnancy, facts mentioned by Dr. Abbott, which undoubtedly increased her symptomatology. The fact that patient still has a significant amount of discomfort in her back would indicate a non-organic basis, as she has a solid spine fusion, which eliminated the alleged instability, and yet patient has continued to complain.

Everett J. Gordon, M.D.

PROGRESS REPORTS

Progress reports should be rendered approximately every two to three weeks, depending on the extent of the patient's injury and his response to therapy. Most cases of cervical and low back strain will respond to proper treatment in four to six weeks. A satisfactory plan is to re-examine the patient after 4 to 6 treatments, generally within the first two weeks, to note his progress and response to treatment. At this point it may be necessary to reinforce the treatment plan by addition of external supports such as a cervical collar or low back support, to supplement the medication or change to a more potent muscle relaxant and analgesic, or to make recommendations or changes for additional physical therapy. It is not advisable to refer the patient to a physical therapist for an extended period of several weeks without periodic check-up and reappraisal of his condition.

Frequently, the patient develops new complaints within a few days of his initial visit, especially when he is first examined immediately after his accident. At this time, many patients report only what hurts the most and pay little attention to areas of less discomfort. After a few days they begin to notice bruises here and there or aching in other parts of the body, frequently the low back area. The patient should report these complaints to the therapist, who should refer him back to his physician for additional examination and x-rays if indicated. The findings should be included in a progress report. A second examination and reappraisal within seven to ten days of the initial visit will result in a more complete and accurate diagnosis and also insure proper treatment.

The patient usually appreciates close supervision by his physician, and this will be reflected in an improved patient-doctor relationship. The doctor should record all of his examinations by dictating progress notes which can be immediately mailed or held in the file, and supplemented periodically. The progress reports can be left open after each dictation, then forwarded at the end of four to six weeks rather than mailed individually. If the case is not closed in four to six weeks, the progress report should be forwarded to the attorney at that time; this report should indicate how much additional treatment is planned and when the patient will be able to return to work.

The following are suggested outlines of progress reports after treatment of injuries to the cervical and lumbar areas. They should be supplemented with information regarding other injuries treated such as the knee, hand, etc. Specific ranges of motion may be measured and reported if necessary to indicate the patient's response to treatment.

Interval Examination

LUMBAR SPINE

Patient has been receiving physical therapy to the low back area in the form of hot packs _____, diathermy _____, medcosonlator _____, massage _____, exercises _____. At this time he _____ she _____ feels improved in response to the treatment given.

ON EXAMINATION: There is an improved range of flexion-extension motion of the lumbar area, with less pain with these motions; also a good range of lateral flexion, right and left with less discomfort.

Treatment will gradually be diminished; physical therapy to be given three times a week, _____ twice a week, _____ for _____ weeks, following which the patient will be re–evaluated.

CERVICAL SPINE

Patient has improved after receiving multiple physical therapy to the cervical spine, upper back and shoulders consisting of hot packs _____, diathermy _____, massage _____, medcosonlator _____, Sayre halter traction _____. At this time, he _____ she _____ has a few _____, no complaints relative to the involved areas but feels improved. He _____ She _____ has _____ has not _____ returned to work as of _____.

ON EXAMINATION: There is an improved range of motion of the cervical spine with less discomfort and muscle spasm, with lateral flexion and rotation, forward flexion and extension. Shoulder motion is satisfactory and performed without undue discomfort. The muscle spasm and tenderness has improved.

Further treatment is indicated in the form of _____ and will be given at intervals of three times a week, _____ twice a week, _____ for _____ weeks, following which patient will be re-evaluated.

Generally, bills are not rendered until after the treatment is complete and they are not forwarded with periodic progress reports. Occasionally, the attorney will request an estimate of the physician's fees for purposes of negotiating with the insurance carrier, and this can be given. If the physician has recommended that therapy will be given over an extended period, he should indicate this in his report to the attorney.

After a patient has been under treatment for several weeks, it is usually a good plan to defer final evaluation for one to two weeks or longer after the last therapy session, in order to better evaluate the patient's progress and response to therapy, and also to check for any relapse in his condition. Occasionally, the patient will wonder why he cannot be discharged at the time of his last treatment, especially if he has no complaints. It should be explained that there may be a relapse or reoccurrence of symptoms after therapy has ceased, and therefore there should be an interim period before the final evaluation is made.

At the time of the last treatment, the patient should be advised of the necessity of returning for a final evaluation. If this is deferred for a month or more, a significant number of these patients will not return as they will forget the appointment, especially if they feel well. Sometimes it is necessary to explain that a final report is required by the attorney in order for him to enter into successful negotiations with the defendant. Generally, a period of one to two weeks is advisable; experience has shown that longer periods result in a high percentage of no returns, requiring letters or phone calls in an effort to close the file. If no residual disability is anticipated, a one-week interval should suffice and will result in a higher percentage of kept appointments.

Should the patient fail to return for the appointment, it is a good practice to send him a card giving him a specific number of days, such as five to seven, to call for an appointment; the cards should also notify him that should he fail to make an appointment within that period, his file will be closed. At that point, the case should be closed by sending the attorney, or insurance carrier in a Workmen's Compensation case, a final note indicating that the patient did not return for follow-up care; a bill should also be submitted with the final report.

A report should be forwarded promptly after the final examination. This should include all pertinent data which the attorney will require to estimate the value of his case, including subjective complaints such as headaches, morning stiffness, nervousness, etc., and objective findings—scars, impaired function, restricted joint motion, muscle atrophy, joint swelling, etc. An opinion should be expressed regarding permanency of the residual findings and an estimate of degree of disability. Date of return to work and work capacity should also be included in a final report. A final bill should accompany this report. If the patient has health and accident insurance, coverage from Blue Shield, or medical pay coverage on his auto, these claims should be prepared and filed, accompanied by properly executed assignments if the bill has not been paid.

The following reports are suggested outlines for individuals who have made a good recovery. Additional information may be added as indicated for each individual case.

FINAL EXAMINATION

CERVICAL

Patient has improved in response to physical therapy given in this office to the cervical _____ and upper dorsal areas. At this time, patient has no _____ relatively few _____ complaints in the injured areas. He/She _____ has/has not _____ returned to work.

ON EXAMINATION: There is a full range of motion in the cervical area, including flexion extension, rotation and lateral bending, with no discomfort produced by these motions. He/She _____ performs a good trapezius shrug without difficulty. Lateral cervical compression causes no radiation to either shoulder. Full range of motion in both shoulders, including lateral abduction, overhead elevation, external internal rotation. Reflexes and sensation are intact in both upper extremities. No tenderness or muscle spasm in the cervical area.

Patient is now being discharged from active care. There is no need of further treatment at the present time. Should there be an exacerbation, patient was advised to return to this office.

LUMBAR

Patient has been treated in this office with hot packs, _____ medcosonlator _____, exercises _____, massage _____ given at regular intervals. At this time patient has no _____ few _____ complaints pertaining to the low back area, and may return _____ has returned_____ to work.

ON EXAMINATION: He/She _____ bends forward without discomfort or restriction. Lateral flexion, torsion, backward extension motions also well performed without difficulty. No tenderness or muscle spasm in the lumbar area. Straight leg raising, Lasègue, and Yeoman hip hyperextension tests are easily performed without difficulty. Patient hyperextends the back against gravity without pain.

At this time, patient appears to have made a satisfactory recovery from the injuries to his/her _____ lower back sustained in the accident of _____ (date). No further treatment is required at this time. However, should patient have any exacerbation of his/her _____ problem, he/she _____ was advised to again contact this office.

CERVICAL AND LUMBAR

Patient has improved in response to physical therapy given in this office to the cervical, upper dorsal and lumbar areas. At this time, he/she _____ has no _____ only a few _____ complaints in the injured areas. He/She _____ has/has not _____ returned to work.

ON EXAMINATION: There is a full range of motion in the cervical area, including flexion extension, rotation and lateral bending, with no discomfort produced by these motions. He/She _____ performs a good trapezius shrug without difficulty. Lateral cervical compression causes no radiation to either shoulder. Full range of motion in both shoulders, including lateral abduction, overhead elevation, external internal rotation. Reflexes and sensation are intact in both upper extremities. No tenderness or muscle spasm in the cervical area.

ON EXAMINATION: Improvement in the lower back. He/She _____ bends forward without discomfort or restriction. Lateral flexion, torsion, backward extension motions also well performed without difficulty. No tenderness or muscle spasm in the lumbar area. Straight leg raising, Lasègue and Yeoman hip hyperextension tests are easily performed without difficulty. Patient hyperextends the back against gravity without pain.

At this time patient appears to have made a satisfactory recovery from the injuries to his/her _____ neck and lower back, sustained in the accident of _____ (date). No further treatment is required at this time. However, should patient have any exacerbation of his/her _____ problem, he/she _____ is advised to again contact this office.

During the course of treatment it is proper for the attorney to request information from the attending physician, to aid him in determining whether a suit should be filed, also to place a settlement value upon the case. In some instances he may request a conference with the doctor, usually scheduled after regular office hours when there will be no interrupting phone calls, or he may suggest that the attending physician outline any further treatment and the anticipated course in a medical report (in either case the physician should make a charge for the additional services). If surgery is anticipated, this should be stated, as well as the doctor's fee, the approximate cost of hospitalization, and the prognosis. However, if there is no true indication or medical basis for surgery, the physician should not discuss the need for surgery and speculate regarding possible poor results merely for the benefit of the attorney.

An orthopaedist who performs frequent defendant examinations occasionally encounters instances of unwarranted surgery and speculative prognoses among the medical reports sent to him for his review prior to the evaluation of a plaintiff. There are very few physicians who engage in this type of activity, and they soon become identified and labeled, with a resultant diminution in their credibility. The doctor who will write what the attorney tells him, loses his value as an expert witness. The judges also recognize this type of individual and place little credence in the opinions he expresses. The cases detailed under "Reports Concerning Surgical Procedures (pp. 152–160) are striking examples of what may occur when a doctor abandons his ethical medical principles to give his full cooperation to an attorney's desire for a strong catastrophic type of prognosis.

AVAILABILITY OF HOSPITAL RECORDS

Occasionally a question arises regarding the availability of hospital records in a medico-legal case. It has long been the custom of hospitals not to release any type of record to attorneys or insurance companies without the prior approval of the physician who treated the patient at the hospital; without that approval the records were not released. However, in the past couple of years most hospitals have been releasing their records upon receipt of proper authorization from the patient or his representative, and simultaneously notifying the attending physician of their action.

In the case of *Emmett* vs *Eastern Dispensary and Casualty Hospital,* No. 396F2D931, in the United States District Court for the District of Columbia, it was held that a patient is absolutely entitled to a copy of his hospital record and that this privilege is extended to his next of kin in the event of the death of the patient. The court further said that the refusal to release such records to a person entitled to them would constitute fraudulent concealment, tolling the statute of limitations. The consent of the attending physician is not required for the release of medical records to the patient or his representative, and any direction by the physician that the record not be released should not be honored, according to this ruling.

The hospital records have always been available by means of a subpoena obtained by either litigant. Thus the records could be made available whether the physician consented or not. However, in order to obtain a subpoena, a suit must be filed first; this can often be avoided if the records are voluntarily offered for the attorney's review. This situation was exemplified by an incident in which the author refused to authorize the hospital to release a patient's chart to her attorney in a minor malpractice claim.

Subsequently, suit was filed and the records were obtained by subpoena. When it was learned that the patient had gone into a definite catatonic state after minor surgery necessitating transfer to a mental hospital, and that she had been an in-patient in that hospital for the two previous years (a fact not reported to the attending physician), the case was quickly settled for a small nuisance sum. Had the plaintiff attorney been permitted to review the patient's chart on his initial request, suit would probably not have been filed, and there would have been no blemish on the physician's insurance record.

REVIEW OF MEDICAL REPORTS FOR DEFENDANT EXAMINATION

A medical specialist who performs frequent defendant examinations is often relied upon to evaluate complicated, difficult cases, which have received extensive periods of treament or had surgery resulting in inadequate relief of the subjective complaints. Some of these patients have been under treatment for two or three years and continue to complain until the time of trial. They have developed thick files of medical reports and a long list of expenses for loss of wages, medical care, hospitalization, braces and medicines, and specialist consultations.

Some medical groups with a large plaintiff practice see the patients at regular weekly intervals, then semi-weekly, and then every four to six weeks during the entire period before the case comes to trial. Stereotyped reports are submitted after each visit or at least monthly. Most of these reports outline the patient's continued subjective complaints and include few objective findings.

Usually these reports are forwarded to the defendant examiner in advance, for his review prior to conducting his examination. It is anticipated that there will be a charge for the time used in the perusal of these reports. It is good practice to abstract these documents in advance, dictating the substance contained in them and pertinent comments, then adding this separately to the reports submitted to the insurance carrier or the defendant's attorney. This review will often provide the examiner with an excellent background of the case and give him a good idea of what to expect when the patient reports to the office.

Time spent in abstracting the medical reports will facilitate the examination, although there is always the chance that the plaintiff will not keep his appointment and the examination will never be performed. However, if the physician has devoted his time to analysis of the reports, he should forward his abstract with a bill for services rendered. This may be of some value to the defendant, even though the time used by the physician for review of records has been essentially wasted, as he has more important use for his professional time.

ALTERATION OF REPORTS

The attorney may request the treating physician to alter the report he has submitted because of factual errors or misleading phraseology; this is a legitimate request which should be granted. However, some attorneys are overly aggressive and frequently request corrections or even suggest the phrasing they desire. If the doctor has made an error, such as a date or location, he should correct it, but he should not change his description of the injuries and diagnoses unless there is a valid medical reason to do so. In particular, he should not delete references to prior accidents, illnesses, or surgery if the patient has informed him of these events and he has recorded them accurately; occasionally the plaintiff attorney makes this type of request because he believes such material diminishes the value of his present claim. If the physician does omit some facts on request, and they become known to the defendant, he may be embarrassed on the witness stand during his cross-examination.

Sometimes there are aspects of the case which irritate either the doctor or the attorney but which can be settled by a conference and discussion of mutual problems. In other instances they can be resolved by a slight adjustment and rephrasing of reports. The doctor may not be aware of the importance of minor phrases in his report which can be of serious import to the attorney who receives it. For example, the doctor should not volunteer a percentage rating after examining the patient for the defendant unless it is specifically requested. In preparing reports for the plaintiff, he should avoid phrases which depreciate the case, but the same meaning can be indicated in his method of treatment. For example, if he does not believe any medication is indicated, he should not prescribe any; it is not necessary to write, "Because of the mildness of the injury, no medication is being ordered." Similarly, if physical therapy is not indicated, it should not be ordered, but a statement should not be made to the effect that "inasmuch as patient has few objective findings, no physical therapy is being ordered." A physician may make such a statement in his report, yet order hot packs or warm tub baths at home; in effect he is providing treatment despite his statement, "Because of the mildness of the injury, no treatment is indicated." The inference is apparent from his method of care.

FORWARDING OF REPORTS

The physician's report of his examination and treatment should only be sent to the party who requested the examination or referred the patient to the doctor. If the patient was referred by an attorney, a signed authorization and assignment form should be secured from the patient and forwarded to his lawyer for acknowledgement and counter-signature, before mailing him any report or bill. Referrals from the defendant insurance company require no written authorization, as the examination has already been authorized by agreement between the plaintiff or his attorney and the defendant. Difficulties sometimes arise when the patient erroneously states that he is appearing for the examination at the request of his attorney, when he is actually being examined on behalf of the defendant, who had instructed the patient's attorney to make the appointment. Reports may be submitted to the wrong party under these circumstances, resulting in possible embarrassment for the examining physician if he has made recommendations for treatment, which is not indicated in a defendant evaluation. These situations may be avoided if the doctor's receptionist questions the source of referral and calls the attorney's office to verify it. Apparent referrals from unfamiliar lawyers are often from defendant insurance companies. If the accident occurred several months or years before the appointment, the examination is more likely to be for the defendant, but not always.

If the plaintiff's attorney asks for a copy of the physician's report which had been sent to the insurance company requesting the examination, the report should not be mailed unless the doctor has specific instructions from the defendant to do so. This may have been authorized in the original memorandum referring the patient for the examination; if permission is granted by telephone, a note should be recorded in the chart with the date and name of the individual who authorized a copy of the report to be mailed to the opposing party.

Although such a request usually originates with the plaintiff attorney, occasionally the treating doctor is contacted by an insurance adjuster for this information, either by telephone or letter. If the patient has not secured legal counsel and is willing to sign a written authorization, a report can be sent to him. Some physicians have the patient sign a blank consent form which is kept in the chart to be used to forward reports to either an attorney or an insurance adjuster, as the patient directs at a later date.

Even though the doctor has a consent form in the file, he should not comply with a request for his report from an insurance company if he has personal knowledge that his patient subsequently employed an attorney, regardless of whether the doctor has received any communications from that attorney. This is true even when the insurance company forwards a properly signed authorization from the patient. He should notify the patient of the request and ask for clarification, as in many instances the patient signed the authorization slip at the initial interview with the adjuster, then reconsidered and contacted an attorney. In most cases, after the patient contacts his attorney, he will direct the physician to ignore the request. By following this procedure, the doctor will preserve his neutral and impartial status, particularly if he happens to perform frequent defense examinations and has personal contacts with many insurance company representatives. Occasionally, a friendly adjuster will try to take advantage of his acquaintance with the doctor and ask for medical information over the telephone *on the QT;* this violates the doctor-patient relationship and the request should be gently refused, with a reminder to his insurance friend that he knows very well that the doctor cannot ethically comply. Usually the request is made because the adjuster cannot obtain a copy of the doctor's medical report from the patient's attorney, who probably has been an uncooperative and a difficult negotiator. The doctor should answer the request for a report by stating he has sent sufficient copies to the other party for distribution as they desire.

A similar problem but with different legal interpretation occasionally occurs with reports of injuries under the Workmen's Compensation law. All reports are sent to the carrier and the doctor is not authorized to send a report to any other party except to the Workmen's Compensation Commission, or possibly to the employer. A request and authorization signed by the patient does not have the same significance in a Workmen's Compensation case as in a private one, as the doctor-patient relationship is different. A third party, the employer, has retained the doctor's services and authorized the treatment, and is paying for it; the records belong to that party or his representative (the Workmen's Compensation Insurance Carrier). Thus, a request for a report from an attorney later employed by the patient should be referred to the insurance carrier. A brief, polite note to the attorney should advise him that you have forwarded several copies of the report to the insurance carrier, and give the name of the adjuster he may contact for further information. Rarely is there any further correspondence on the subject. If the attorney is knowledgeable, he will realize the doctor is aware of his legal responsibilities and is correct in his answer. The information is also available to him through the file maintained at the regional Workmen's Compensation Commission office. Occasionally, however, the attorney will phone the doctor and threaten him with a subpoena to obtain the records. In such cases, he should contact the insurance carrier and request that they contact the attorney, or he may obtain advice and guidance from the regional industrial commission.

Medical reports of disability evaluations performed for the United States Civil Service Commission cannot be forwarded to the patient, his attorney, or other agencies despite a signed authorization from the patient. This information is rigidly protected by the Civil Service Commission regulations; their express permission must be secured before release of any information.

5 FEES

THE PHYSICIAN IS ENTITLED TO PAYMENT FOR HIS PROFESSIONAL SERVICES WHICH INCLUDE EXAMINATION AND TREATMENT, PREPARATION OF MEDICO-LEGAL REPORTS, CONFERENCES WITH ATTORNEYS, COURT TESTIMONY, REVIEW OF RECORDS AND X-RAYS, AND RESEARCH AND PREPARATION FOR TRIAL. HE IS NOT EXPECTED TO RENDER EXTRAORDINARY SERVICES BEYOND THE NORMAL SCOPE OF MEDICAL CARE WITHOUT COMPENSATION.

FEE SCHEDULES

The physician's fees charged for these services should be fair and in keeping with those rendered by other physicians of similar standing in his own community. In Workmen's Compensation cases there is usually an established fee schedule approved by the local Medical Society to which the physician should adhere, although deviations are permitted for exceptional cases or services not listed in the schedule, such as review of hospital records, review of x-rays at hospitals, conferences with attorneys, unusual surgical procedures, etc.

The fee for a detailed medico-legal examination and report is usually greater than that charged for orthopaedic consultation for diagnostic and therapeutic purposes alone. The charge reflects the additional time necessary in a medico-legal case for a more detailed examination and preparation of a complex report, which must be accomplished with care if it is to be of value to the interested party.

The usual fee for the preparation of medico-legal reports varies from twenty-five to thirty-five dollars, as suggested by the Orange County, California Medical Association,[29] which published a guide for determining fees for physicians' services in medico-legal cases in May 1969. The guide also suggests fees for review of hospital records, deposition and testimony, the latter varying from 200 to 250 dollars for a half-day of a court appearance. It is also noted that if the court appointment was cancelled less than twenty-four hours in advance, a fee of one-half of the agreed amount should be paid. The doctor should not be hesitant in mentioning a fee for the additional work involved when an attorney or insurance company requests a medical report concerning a patient whom he has had under treatment. Many will include a statement in their request that they anticipate a bill for the additional services requested, but it may be wise to inform the attorney or insurance company as to the amount of the fee, so that there will be no disagreement once the report and your bill have been received.

The physician should charge his regular fee for office visits, injections, physical therapy, and so forth, but additional charges for check-up examinations and progress reports are usual and accepted. Under no circumstances should the doctor "pad" his bill because it is a medico-legal case; if he does, he will ultimately face considerable embarrassment on the witness stand, and his stature will certainly be diminished in the community when other physicians and attorneys became aware of this undesirable practice.

A copy of the bill for professional services rendered constitutes an essential part of the medico-legal report and should accompany the final report submitted to the patient's attorney or defendant insurance carrier. The bill should be carefully itemized with dates for each service rendered. A lump sum is ordinarily not acceptable and will probably be questioned in court. Separate charges for reports are not compensable by the defendant; if testimony is given regarding fees, any charge for reports should be deleted from the total bill for professional medical services. The doctor may also bill the patient for pre-trial conferences with the attorney, but again this portion of the bill cannot be submitted to the defendant.

At the time the case is closed, copies of the bill should be sent to the patient, as well as to the attorney, so the former will be aware of his responsibility and obligation. This is in accordance with the physician's position that his fee is not subject to contingency, in contrast to the patient's agreement with his attorney. Otherwise, the patient will believe that his bill is being taken care of by his attorney and that he has no responsibility; this belief must be quickly dispelled, in accordance with approved medical ethics. Notations on the bill for information of settlement of the case is helpful while waiting for payment from the attorney.

ASSIGNMENTS

A physician is never permitted to charge on a contingent basis, dependent upon successful recovery in the lawsuit; his bill must be independent of the outcome of the case. The attorney usually takes the case on a contingency basis, but for the physician to take this position would be unethical and unlawful as it would encourage false and exaggerated testimony and suppression of the truth. However, it is both proper and prudent to have the patient sign an assignment and authorization form; as a matter of fact, many of these have been standardized and jointly approved by medical and legal associations in various communities. The form will authorize the doctor to forward his report to the attorney, and also will permit the attorney to deduct sufficient money from whatever recovery is made to pay any fees that have not already been paid by the patient prior to final disposition of the case. The attorney should demonstrate his cooperation with the physician by acknowledging receipt of the form with his counter signature.[12]

The following assignment forms were devised by the author in conjunction with representatives of the local Bar Association, and are in general use in the District of Columbia. (They may be reproduced without permission.)

A. For Attorney

Three copies of this form are to be signed by the patient on the initial visit. No figures can be stated as the final amount of the medical bill is unknown, but if the patient wishes, the physician may insert: "Not to exceed $_____." It is important that it be signed initially as the patient may not return after the first visit and this may be the only means by which the physician can collect his bill through the patient's attorney. If the patient does not proceed with his litigation, the cost of the form is negligible and it can be discarded. One copy is retained in the patient's chart and two copies are sent to his attorney for his counter signature and acceptance of the assignment. The attorney returns one copy to the doctor and retains one copy in his file. The completed form containing the attorney's signature is photostated and a copy sent to the patient for his information, so that he will have a copy of what he has signed. In addition, the last two sentences are underlined to emphasize his personal responsibility for the bill.

ASSIGNMENT AND AUTHORIZATION†
(Form No. I)

I, _____, hereby authorize my physician, *Everett J. Gordon, M. D., 730 24th Street, N.W., Washington, D.C.,* to furnish my attorney _____ Esq., and/or _____ Insurance Company, any medical reports which he or they may request in reference to the injuries sustained by me, my wife or children on _____.

I further authorize and direct said attorney or insurance company to pay from the proceeds of any recovery in my case to my physician, *Everett J. Gordon, M. D.,* for his professional services (including children, as a result of the injuries heretofore mentioned. I understand that this in no way relieves me of my personal primary responsibility to pay my physician for such services when statement is rendered. It is understood that the signing of this form does not prohibit customary billing.

NAME: _____

Address: _____

WITNESS: _____   Date: _____

The undersigned attorney for the patient referred to herein above hereby agrees to comply fully with the foregoing "Assignment and Authorization" and agrees to advise the named doctor in writing within ten days of his request for information regarding the status of the claim of the aforesaid patient.

Date: _____   _____Esq.

ATTORNEY Signature

*** ATTORNEY: Please date, sign and return one copy of this agreement to the doctor's office. Medical reports will be forwarded upon its *receipt*. Keep one copy for your records.

†THIS form has been approved and sanctioned by both the District of Columbia Medical Society and the District of Columbia Bar Association.

An alternative form has recently been devised which emphasizes the personal liability of the patient for the physician's bill and also tolls the statute of limitations.

ASSIGNMENT AND AUTHORIZATION

I, _____, hereby authorize my physician, *Everett J. Gordon, M. D., 730 24th St. N.W. Washington, D.C., 20037,* to furnish my attorney _____, Esq., and/or _____ Insurance Company, any medical reports which he or they may request in reference to the injuries sustained by me, my wife, or children on _____.

I further authorize and direct said attorney or insurance company to deduct and pay from the proceeds of any recovery in my case, or any monies which they may receive on my behalf in connection with my claim for damages for personal injury to my physician, *Everett J. Gordon, M.D.,* for his professional services (including fees for preparation and testimony) to myself, my wife or my children, as a result of the injuries heretofore mentioned. I authorize this sum to be paid directly to *Dr. Gordon* at the time compensatory monies are received. I understand that this in no way relieves me of my personal primary responsibility to pay my physician for such services when statement is rendered. It is understood that the signing of this form does not prohibit customary billing.

I also understand that if favorable legal settlement does not occur, I remain personally liable for payment of the total bill for professional services rendered to me by *Dr. Everett J. Gordon.*

I hereby agree to waive the defense of the statute of limitations; in the event that a claim is filed against me by reason of any unpaid bill, I will no raise the defense of the statute of limitations.

NAME: _____

Address: _____

WITNESS: _____   Date: _____

I, the undersigned attorney for the patient referred to herein above hereby agrees to comply fully with the foregoing "Assignment and Authorization" and agree TO ADVISE THE NAMED DOCTOR IN WRITING WITHIN TEN DAYS OF HIS REQUEST FOR IN-FORMATION REGARD THE STATUS OF THE CLAIM OF THE AFORESAID PATIENT. I ALSO AGREE TO NOTIFY THE DOCTOR IMMEDIATELY OF ANY CHANGE IN THE STATUS OF THIS CASE WHICH MAY PRECLUDE PAYMENT OF HIS PROFESSIONAL FEE BY THIS OFFICE.

Date: _____Esq.

ATTORNEY SIGNATURE

*** ATTORNEY: Please date, sign and return one copy of this agreement to the doctor's office. Medical reports will be forwarded upon its *receipt*. Keep one copy for your records.

B. For Medical Pay Coverage

Two copies of this form are signed by the the patient if he indicates that he has medical pay coverage on his own vehicle, or if he is not represented by counsel and wishes to negotiate directly with the insurance company. It also may be substituted for the preceding forms to be sent to the attorney, if a limited dollar value of the assignment is desirable. At the conclusion of treatment, one copy is kept in the file and the other copy forwarded with the reports and bill to the patient's own insurance carrier if a medical pay claim has been made, or to the insurance carrier of the defendant, if he has no attorney and authorizes this procedure. The insurance adjuster should be contacted in advance by phone or letter for assurance that he will honor the assignment and include the doctor's name on the settlement check or pay the doctor directly.

ASSIGNMENT AND AUTHORIZATION†

(Form No. 2)

This is to authorize and direct my attorney _____Esq. and/or _____ Insurance Company to receive all medical reports and to pay directly my physician, Everett J. Gordon, M.D., 730 24th Street, N.W., Washington, D.C., his bill in the sum of, or not to exceed _____

Dollars ($_____) or balance thereof, representing a fair and

just charge for professional services rendered _____;
said payment to be made from any monies received by said attorney
or insurance company as a result of settlement or action on my
claim, or medical pay coverage, because of injuries received by
_____ on or about _____.
Payment of this amount as herein directed, in whole or part, shall
be the same as if paid by me. It is further agreed that nothing
herein contained relieves me of the primary responsibility and obligation of paying my physician, Everett J. Gordon, M.D., his fee for
medical services when statement is rendered. It is understood that
the signing of this form does not prohibit customary billing.

                          NAME: _____

                          Address: _____

WITNESS: _____ Date: _____

    The undersigned attorney for the patient referred to herein
above hereby agrees to comply fully with the foregoing "Assignment and Authorization" and agrees to advise the named doctor in
writing within ten days of his request for information regard the
writing within ten days of his request for information regarding the
status of the claim of the aforesaid patient.

Date: _____ _____Esq.

                     ATTORNEY Signature

***   ATTORNEY: Please date, sign and return one copy of this agree-
             ment to the doctor's office. Medical reports will be
             forwarded upon its *receipt*. Keep one copy for your
             records.

    It should be clearly understood by the patient that the doc-
tor's fees are not contingent upon anticipated recovery, and the
assignment does not relieve the patient of his primary responsibility to pay his physician. Otherwise he may be under the impression that the doctor has the same financial arrangement as
the contingency agreement signed with his attorney. The patient
should also be notified that payment is expected within a reasonable time, although the doctor may be willing to cooperate with
the attorney and wait for resolution of the case if not too prolonged.

    Frequently, however, payment must await a successful re-
covery as the patient either has no financial resources or he does
not believe he is obligated to make payment out of his own
pocket. This belief may have been encouraged by the attorney
who often tells the patient "not to worry about payment as I

will take care of it." The patient then feels that he has no obligation to the doctor, even though the assignment forms clearly state otherwise. In all cases the patient should be regularly billed and payment obtained prior to resolution of the case wherever possible.

Reports are usually sent to the patient's attorney after receipt of the properly signed agreement forms, even though payment has not been received. A few physicians make a practice to inform the patients and their attorneys that they will not send any reports until payment has been received; this may be a good policy to adopt if the patient appears to be unreliable and the doctor is unfamiliar with the attorney's reputation.

PERIODIC STATUS REPORTS

The physician who has been active in medico-legal practice will soon accumulate a considerable backlog of cases in litigation with unpaid medical fees. Although he should bill these patients on a regular basis, it will become necessary to wait for resolution of a large percentage of these cases. The physician is often placed in a position of major dependency upon the plaintiff's attorney to obtain payment for him when a recovery is made. Thus, it is expedient for the physician to contact the plaintiff attorney at regular intervals, at least once every six months, by letter or telephone, to learn the status of the pending litigation. He should mark his records accordingly, so that he will be current with the developments in the case. Most attorneys will notify the physician if they no longer represent the patient or if unforeseen circumstances develop which preclude recovery, but there are always a few who neglect to inform the doctor that he can no longer look to them for payment because of an unsuccessful termination of the case. The client may change lawyers, or move to another city, he may become incarcerated, or investigation may prove that there is no insurance on the other vehicle and there is no chance of recovery from the uninsured driver. Some individuals become involved in accidents and are treated by physicians in the emergency room, then disappear. In some instances the case may have been tried and lost without the physician's knowledge, as he was not called as a witness.

Of course the attorney should notify the doctor when any of these incidents occur, but sometimes he does not do so because of the pressure of his practice and lack of methodical habits. The physician will have little chance of recovery of his fees in those cases in which there is a considerable time lapse. Attorneys who value the physician's services usually notify the physician of such a change in status of his case, but many busy, reputable attorneys forget that the physician is dependent upon them for recovery of his fee. Thus it becomes necessary for the physician to protect his accounts receivable involving medico-legal cases by regularly contacting the attorneys to learn their current status.

A form letter has been devised for this purpose and is quite effective, but it is necessary to follow up these letters with telephone calls, as approximately one-third of the attorneys do not answer the initial written inquiry. However, repeated phone calls usually secure the necessary information. The following letter has been found to be useful:

> Would you please set forth the status of the following cases in which our records indicate that you are the attorney? Your cooperation would be appreciated and will facilitate the continued handling of this type of case by our office. An addressed envelope is enclosed for your convenience.
>
> If no reply is received from you by _____, it will be assumed that you are no longer representing this individual and the patient will be contacted directly for further investigation and payment.
>
> I hope you will give this your prompt attention in order to avoid further correspondence and phone calls which will require additional time of both your office and mine. You can be assured of my continued cooperation if you will take the few minutes necessary to complete and return this form. Please use the reverse side if necessary.
>
> Everett Gordon, M.D.

NAME	STATUS

This request for information does not represent an unjust imposition upon the attorney, as the physician has cooperated with him by waiting for settlement of the litigation, and the time required for answering this form is minimal. Cooperation between the two professions in this manner will result in a favorable and improved business relationship between the medical and legal professions. When the attorney fails to notify the physician of an important change, such as the fact that he no longer represents the client or has transferred the case to another jurisdiction, the harmonious relationship becomes disrupted and occasionally leads to bitter conflict between the two professions.

Such an incident occurred in *Gibson* vs *Heffelfinger,* in which the attorney forwarded the case to an attorney in another jurisdiction where he was not licensed to practice. The physician was not aware of the change of status of the case and apparently his unpaid account lay dormant in the file for many years. Approximately five years after treatment of the patient, he learned that the case had been settled and disbursement made to the patient without protection of his bill. He was able to collect only half of his bill from the patient, following which he brought suit against the initial attorney for collection of the balance of his medical fees, in accordance with a properly signed assignment, which did not obligate the second attorney.

In the subsequent action brought by the treating physician against the attorney who initially represented the patient, an opinion was rendered in favor of the physician, requiring the attorney to pay the balance of the medical fees which had not been paid by the patient. This situation could have been avoided had the attorney protected the physician's fee when he forwarded the case to his correspondent attorney. In addition, he should have notified the physician that he was no longer actively representing the client, and that the physician should contact the new attorney, who would assume the responsibility for the litigation and distribution of any money recovered therefrom. A short letter would have avoided the embarrassment and expense of the lawsuit that ensued, and the verdict against the defendant attorney. (*Gibson* vs *Heffelfinger,* No. GS18233-70, Superior Court, D. C., 99 *Washington* Law Reporter 1393). (Heffelfinger vs. Gibson, #290-A-20-390; D. C. Court of Appeals 4/21/72. A.M.A. Citation, Vol. 26, No. 4, 12/1/72, pp. 62–63.)

HEALTH AND ACCIDENT INSURANCE—ASSIGNMENTS

If the patient has a health and accident insurance policy which will reimburse him for the doctor's services, the proceeds should be assigned to the doctor and applied to his bill, thus leaving a smaller balance to be paid by the attorney at the time of recovery. If the benefits are principally for loss of time from work or disability payments, this may be assigned to the doctor or paid to the patient in hardship cases. Occasionally the patient will wish to collect the proceeds of his accident policy for medical services, believing that the doctor should wait for settlement of his litigation. This would be grossly unfair as the patient would then collect for the doctor's services, but the doctor would remain unpaid. The case may require several years for resolution and could result in an unfavorable final decision. This should be explained to the patient; if he still is reluctant to sign the assignment forms, the doctor should call the attorney and explain his position. If the attorney declines to cooperate, then the physician should reconsider whether he wishes any further relationships with that particular attorney except on a *pay as you go* basis. He may also decline to complete the insurance forms payable to the patient until his bill is paid in full.

Insurance payment orders similar to the following should be signed by the patient on the initial visit, to be used for assignment of any benefits due from health and accident plans other than Aetna Government-Wide plan or Blue Shield plan, which already have assignments associated with their form. Personal health and accident forms often pay for x-rays, office visits, arthrocentesis of joint, casts, minor surgery, fractures, etc., but some plans do not pay for physical therapy. All payments received should be applied to the patient's account while awaiting settlement of his litigation.

ASSIGNMENT OF BENEFITS

Date _____

TO: _____
(Insurance Company)

_____
(Address)

Group No. _____ Certificate No. _____

I hereby authorize that payment of the amount due in my pending claim be made directly to:

EVERETT J. GORDON, M.D.
730 24th St. N.W.
Washington, D. C. 20037

_____

Telephone: (202) 337-0123

Payment is authorized upon your receipt of an itemized statement for services rendered to:

_____
(Name of Patient)

I understand that I am financially responsible for charges not covered by this authorization.

_____
(Signature of Policy Owner)

_____   _____
(Witness)   (Date)

Health and accident policies may be used to pay expenses even if the expenses are covered by a medical pay clause in the plaintiff's automobile policy. The patient pays the premium for such coverage and is entitled to recover unless there is a specific clause prohibiting multiple recovery without reimbursement. For example, Blue Shield and Blue Cross membership can be utilized without interference with payment from other sources. However, if the patient was injured in the course of his employment and the Workmen's Compensation insurance carrier has made payment in his case, the carrier will request reimbursement should there be a third party recovery. Usually, however, the Workmen's Compensation carrier will not pay for the extensive medico-legal reports sent to the patient's attorney. In addition their payment for the services rendered is in accordance with the approved Workmen's Compensation fee schedule, which may be below the prevailing fee schedule for private practice; their payment may leave a balance due which must be paid either by the patient at the time the services are rendered or from the litigation at the time of recovery. The plaintiff's attorney should be kept informed of any such payments and the balance due.

Some Blue Shield plans provide supplemental coverage, such as for government employees or major medical plans in private employment. These plans provide reimbursement of 80 per cent of the medical expenses above a deductible amount. This can be of considerable aid in reducing the patient's indebtedness to the physician prior to conclusion of the litigation.

The physician should utilize an assignment form for payment of supplemental benefits directly to him whenever possible. If the patient is sent an itemized bill, and he is a government employee, he may present that bill under his own supplemental plan; payment will be made directly to him without the physician's knowledge, as the claim form does not require the physician's signature. Those in private employment having a major medical plan require the physician's signature on the claim form and thus the physician would be aware of the application for those benefits. In the case of the government worker, however, it is not uncommon for him to collect these benefits and retain the money for his own use; the physician is then told he must wait until his case is settled before he is paid.

As the purpose of the plan is to *reimburse* the patient for medical expenses (not *pay him* for having become ill), it is not fair to the physician if the patient retains the money for his own use, as he has not expended any of his own funds. It is wise to send only a non-itemized bill if the patient is known to have this type of insurance coverage, and ask him to sign a proper assignment form to permit Blue Shield to pay the doctor directly.

Almost all government workers who have Blue Shield coverage have a supplemental benefit claim provision in their policy, but many have never used it and do not realize that it can be utilized in their personal injury claim. Some private Blue Shield policies from large companies also have a Major Medical claim provision. This form provides an explanation of their benefits:

"If you have Blue Cross and Blue Shield insurance coverage through the Government, you may be eligible for a Supplemental Benefits Claim. This is also true with other plans under Medical Service of the District of Columbia, if you have Major Medical coverage. To obtain such reimbursement, you must obtain a supplemental coverage claim form as the doctor does not have these particular forms. These may be obtained by you either at work from Personnel or by calling Blue Cross and Blue Shield at 484-9000. Ask for the form and when you obtain the form, complete it, sign it and forward to this office. We will then submit this form for you together with an assignment signed by you which will permit the payment to be applied to your account.

"If your account is already paid by other sources, such as medical payment insurance on your car, the money will be refunded to you. The payment is based on 80 per cent reimbursement above your deductible amount. Even if you do not obtain a payment at this time, the claim will be used to offset your deductible amount and later in the year this may be helpful if you have additional medical expense. You will then be able to obtain 80 per cent reimbursement payment after satisfying the deductible. Those who are not in the Government, but have Major Medical Coverage follow a similar policy."

The doctor should secure an assignment of Supplemental Benefits when applicable to the patient's Blue Shield policy, to be signed by *the insured employee* (may be husband or wife or parent of patient) and submit it after completion of treatment, together with a signed Supplemental Benefits claim form. This will pay eighty per cent of the usual and customary medical fees above the deductible (usually one hundred dollars) for office examinations, physical therapy; basic benefits will pay for x-rays, consultations, examinations, physical therapy; basic benefits will pay for x-rays, arthrocentesis, treatment of fractures, minor and major surgery. Funds received through this assignment should be applied to the account while awaiting settlement.

Aetna Government-Wide benefit plan form should be assigned to the doctor by signing where indicated. If the patient is other than the enrollee, the birth date of the enrollee (parent or spouse) must be obtained and entered on the form. This information should be noted on the patient's chart to avoid delays in submission of the form. The plan has a 50 dollar deductible, above which it pays 80 per cent of the customary fees. There are no basic direct benefits available under this plan.

AUTHORIZATION FOR ASSIGNMENT OF BENEFITS

I, _____

(Name of Patient)   (Identification Number)

_____, enrolled under the Govern-

(Name of Federal Employee)

ment Wide Service Benefit Plan, authorize and request Group Hospitalization, Inc., Operations Center to pay to _____

(Name of Provider of Services or Supplies)

Address: _____

Benefits which may be due me for covered services and supplies rendered the patient identified above.

I understand that this authorization applies to those eligible charges submitted with the attached claim incurred in connection with services or supplies furnished only by or through the above Provider, and does not constitute an authorization for assignment of future payments.

I also understand that the Benefits check and a copy of the Benefit Summary form will be mailed directly to the Assignee.

_____   _____

(Date of Authorization)   (Signature of Federal Employee)

Patients often have insurance for disability income while off work as a result of an accident. Some of these forms are relatively simple but still require a certain time for completion. If a detailed form must be submitted, the physician is entitled to charge a minimal fee for the service performed. These payments should not be assigned to the doctor as they are for loss of wages and not reimbursement for medical expenses.

In order to explain more fully to the patient his insurance benefits, a memorandum may be devised and handed to the patient for his information and guidance. Verbal explanations are frequently forgotten or confused and no action is taken.

MEDICAL PAY COVERAGE

If the patient has medical pay coverage in his own insurance policy, this can be used to pay the physician's fee prior to the final disposition of the case. Many policies will pay medical expenses regardless of the outcome of the lawsuit, but some companies have a subrogation clause which provides for their reimbursement if the claimant recovers the money from the defendant. A separate assignment form should be signed by the patient and forwarded with the final bill and report to the medical pay carrier; this enables the physician to be paid directly without unreasonable delay. In most instances the plaintiff's attorney will cooperate with the physician and secure early payment of his client's medical bill, as it is to his advantage to have a cooperative physician if the case must be tried. It is also helpful to his cause if the physician can testify that his bill has already been paid, as sometimes inferences are made by the defendant's attorney that the physician's testimony is prejudiced if he has not been paid prior to trial, suggesting that payment is contingent upon its outcome.

The information for medical pay coverage should be secured from the patient at this first visit or shortly thereafter, noting the name and address of the policy holder and his policy number. If he has already submitted a claim, the claim number will be most helpful. This will enable quicker identification by the carrier and facilitate payment. The claim should be submitted to the regional claims office in the proper jurisdiction; if possible the claim should be addressed to the adjuster handling the claim. It should be noted that some of the larger insurance carriers have several offices in a large metropolitan area, each serving a different business area. If the patient has an identification card stating the name of the insurance agent, the correct office can be identified from the agent or the claim can be forwarded to the agent for transmittal to the proper claims office.

Most patients do not understand the full value of their comprehensive automobile insurance policy. Many have medical pay coverage, but do not know when or how to use it. Their attorney may not discuss this coverage with them as some attorneys believe that the case is diminished in value if they submit a claim for medical payment before the litigation is concluded. They fear the defendant insurance company may obtain a copy of the medical reports in advance through the medical pay carrier, or the demand for payment of special damages will be reduced by the amount paid under medical pay coverage. Occasionally, both the plaintiff and the defendant are insured by the same company and the plaintiff attorney does not wish to create a problem by submission of a medical pay claim.

Because of the recently publicized cancellations of automobile policies, some individuals are apprehensive and fear loss of their coverage because of such a payment, and do not wish to submit a bill or report to their own carrier, in order to reduce the number of accident cases on their record. However, their insurance policy requires them to report all such accidents, and failure to do so may, in itself, cause cancellation of their contract. Payment of justified medical expenses has not been known to cause cancellation of an automobile insurance policy.

However, the medical pay provision is important for the physician as it provides immediate payment without waiting for the litigation to be completed. The authorization and assignment forms for Medical Pay should be signed on the first visit and left in the chart for possible use after treatment has been completed.

The statement below provides the patient with an explanation of his benefits which he can take home and read. As noted previously, explanation requires time and many will not understand or remember verbal information given in the office.

If you have *medical pay* coverage on your automobile insurance you may use it to pay your doctor's bills, also any bills incurred in a hospital emergency room, x-rays, etc. Many companies permit payment from your own policy for medical expenses without reimbursement should you recover from a third party law suit; this means that you may legally recover twice, once from your own company (for which you pay the premium) and also from the party that struck you, if the other party is found at fault. A few companies have what is called a "subrogation clause" which means that they must be reimbursed should you recover from a third party. This does not prevent you from using your insurance to pay your doctor who may not be willing to wait for settlement of your case.

Use of your medical pay coverage permits immediate payment of your bill to the physician, which insures his further co-operation should his services be required at trial. It also may provide additional revenue to you without jeopardizing your own case. This does not prevent you from also using health and accident coverage, which may contribute some payment towards your medical expenses, depending upon the type of coverage you have. It is suggested that you inquire of your own insurance agent regarding multiple coverage.

In all instances *it is necessary for you to submit a proof of claim form to your own insurance carrier* before they will pay your medical costs. *You can obtain such a form from your insurance agent or from the company itself.* This must be completed (and in some instances notarized) before they will consider payment of your medical bills. If in doubt, you may discuss this with your attorney, but it is suggested you take immediate action. Most policies limit payment for only those medical expenses incurred within one year of date of the accident.

This office will be glad to assist you in this matter and will forward your claim for payment. Should you desire your attorney to process this claim, there may be a fee, consistent with your signed agreement with him.

It is suggested you obtain the form without delay and bring it to this office; we will submit your claim when treatment is complete, thus facilitating prompt action. Claim forms for your health and accident insurance should also be secured, completed and signed, then sent to this office for completion of the medical report section. Benefits vary with each insurance company, but most companies will make at least a partial payment for our professional services.

FALSE INFORMATION REGARDING ATTORNEY REPRESENTATION

Before becoming extensively involved in a case requiring x-rays and detailed medical reports, the doctor should discreetly inquire whether the patient is able to pay his bill, either through an attorney who will protect his medical fees by assignment, or through the patient's health and accident insurance, or from personal funds. This is particularly true in a marginal type of case where the patient suffers minor injuries and is apparently exaggerating his complaints, or where liability is dubious, such as in a slip-and-fall case in the grocery store. Sometimes the patient will tell the doctor that he is being represented by an attorney with whom he is familiar; the doctor will assume that the patient has already established a written client-attorney relationship, but this may not be true. In cases of doubt the doctor's secretary should call the attorney to confirm his representation of that patient and to learn if the attorney will protect the doctor's fee. In the so-called *slip-and-fall* cases, such as slipping on a vegetable in a supermarket, the doctor should be particularly suspicious of liability and definite arrangements should be made for payment on a regular basis by the patient. Many of these cases are dropped by the attorney upon receiving the doctor's unfavorable medical report, or are lost in court if they go to trial.

The physician should not permit the referring attorney to use his services to screen potential negligence cases in order to determine whether the attorney will accept the case, unless he is assured of payment for the medical service performed. If the attorney does not return an assignment form with his counter signature within a week, the secretary should phone the attorney to learn the reason. Usually it is because of the attorney's neglect, but occasionally the attorney may inform the doctor that he has never been contacted by the patient and has no intention of representing the patient. He may have represented him in the past and the patient merely used his name. In such cases, the attorney should immediately have contacted the physician upon receipt of the assignment form, but there are many attorneys who are busy or disorganized in their offices, and are not prompt in making even one phone call.

In one incident, a foreign-born patient who had previously been represented by an attorney and had been treated by the same physician, returned two years later after another accident, accompanied by two of his friends involved in the same accident. They gave the name of the previous attorney, which was accepted as the other case had been favorably resolved, and the patients were placed under treatment. Three weeks later, when the assignments had not been returned by the attorney, a phone call revealed that the patients had never contacted that attorney and apparently intended to negotiate their own settlement with the insurance company.

Insurance adjusters will frequently make a nominal settlement without a doctor's report, particularly if the doctor has furnished the patient with a bill. The doctor should become suspicious when a bill is requested under such circumstances, and ask the patient if a settlement is being contemplated. He should request immediate payment to protect his interest and offer to provide a receipted bill, as once settlement is made, it is unlikely that he will ever be paid. No bill was given in this particular case, but it was later learned that the three patients accepted a small settlement from the insurance adjuster, then skipped town.

BILLING PROCEDURE

The fee for a detailed medico-legal examination and report is usually greater than that charged for orthopaedic consultation for diagnostic and therapeutic purposes alone. The charge reflects the additional time necessary for a detailed examination and preparation of a medico-legal report, which must be accomplished with care if it is to be of value to the interested party.

The patient should be billed on a regular basis and partial

payments are requested if he is unable to pay in full. In some cases, however, the patient may inform the doctor of his limited economic assets and request the doctor to wait for settlement. This may be agreeable if the patient's attorney is of good repute and known to be dependable.

The physician should charge his regular fee for office visits, injections, physical therapy, etc., but additional charges for check-up examinations and progress reports are usual and accepted. It cannot be too much emphasized, however, that under no circumstances should the doctor pad his bill because it is a medico-legal case, as he will risk embarrassment before his peers and—we noted this earlier—in the eyes of the community.

A copy of the bill for professional services rendered consti-tutes an essential part of the medico-legal report and should accompany the final report submitted to the patient's attorney or defendant insurance carrier. The bill should be carefully itemized with dates for each service rendered. A lump sum is ordinarily not acceptable and will probably be questioned in court. Separate charges for reports are not compensable by the defen-dant and should be enumerated if questioned; if testimony is given regarding fees, such charges should be deleted from the total bill for professional medical services. The doctor may also bill the patient for pre-trial conferences with the attorney, but again this portion of the bill cannot be submitted to the de-fendant.

DETERMINATION OF FEES FOR TESTIMONY

The charges should in no way be related to the extent of recovery, but should represent a fair and reasonable fee for ser-vices rendered, coresponding to the usual medical fees plus the additional medico-legal services. It is the practice of some medical experts to charge a high or exorbitant fee in medico-legal cases where there are hopes of a large recovery, but this should be condemned. Again, such a policy will lead to the exposure to questioning and general humiliation of the physician in court, deflation of his testimony, and an inevitable loss of community respect. Exorbitant fees for proposed testimony are sometimes quoted to the patient's attorney in the hope they will "price themselves out of the courtroom," but this is unfair to the injured patient whose recovery is often dependent upon the full cooperation of his doctor.

The physician should charge for time involved in pre-trial conferences with the lawyer, review of medical literature associated with the lawsuit, and any other imposition upon his professional time. The fee for testimony depends upon the distance traveled to appear in court, the length of time away from the office, and prevailing fees of similar specialists in that community. Usually there is a gradation in the fee charged for appearing in a court of lower standing than a federal court; the lower courts usually deal with less serious injuries and the proceedings require less time. However, the physician's charge is based primarily upon the amount of time spent in court and on any inconvenience to his practice, including time lost due to the law's delay— recesses, bench conferences, waiting to be called to the stand, and so forth. A fair method of computation is to charge by the hour consistent with the gross income averaged in the physician's practice.[4,8,29]

Some doctors are reluctant to discuss fees for services such as a deposition or testimony. However, it is wise to have a definite understanding in advance with the attorney requesting the doctor's services in order to avoid later difficulties. Often the lawyer will advise the doctor that there is no doubt that he will be paid, as there is clear liability in the case, the defendant is well insured, etc. However, there are many unpredictable factors which often arise and change the entire aspect of the case, such as the death of the defendant, defendant suddenly leaving the country, or other unexpected events, any one of which may jeopardize or delay a favorable resolution of the case. If the doctor has reason to be skeptical of payment at a later date, then he should insist upon payment in full before the taking of his deposition or before giving testimony, or at least have an assignment to be paid at the time the service is rendered.

Although the client is responsible for payment of the fee for medical testimony, the attorney has the responsibility to secure the medical services which are necessary for successful resolution of his case. Some attorneys consider the need for a medical witness as an expense of litigation and advance the sum in the name of their client and charge it to his account. In some instances the doctor will accept a written guarantee from the attorney insuring his fee, to be paid by the attorney regardless of the outcome of the case. Dr. Kent L. Brown of Cleveland discussed this problem at a medico-legal symposium in Miami in May 1967. He observed that the attorney who guarantees payment satisfied the demands of the physician and complied with the requirements of the Canons of Professional Ethics of the American Bar Association. He also noted that it was the attorney's problem whether or not he was reimbursed by his client.[4]

A facet of court testimony which is difficult to resolve is the loss of time for scheduled court appearances which are cancelled or postponed just before the trial. There are many postponements and delays of trials for various reasons beyond the control of the attorney, such as failure of a previous trial to be completed at the anticipated time, absence of witnesses, illnesses of the plaintiff or defendant attorney, of judge or of jurors, mistrials for various reasons which occur before the physician has testified, and others. Attorneys cannot control the court calendar and they too are frustrated by such delays. Another example of what can happen to cause a substantial loss of professional time is the instance when the litigants reach a compromise and settlement just before the trial begins, often as the result of a pre-trial conference in the judge's chambers, or as the outcome of the plaintiff's apprehension when he is faced with actual court proceedings.

If this occurs, the physician's testimony is no longer needed, and he then has a large void in his working day, especially if the trial was to be held in another city and he has cancelled out an entire day from his practice. The doctor has no product, only his professional services, utilizing his time and ability for equal monetary compensation. After he has cancelled office appointments and hospital surgery, he cannot fully recapture his professional time, as usually he is unable to utilize time suddenly made available because of unexpected court action. Although it is generally agreed that the physician is entitled to charge for the interval reserved for testimony, this practice is not always accepted by the patient or his attorney, or even the defendant; any compensation received under these circumstances is usually less than the fee that would have been charged for testimony had it been given. This is of particular concern to the solo practitioner who must necessarily block off valuable appointment time in order to appear in court.

Sometimes the physician does appear in court but his testimony is not given because the case was just settled, or the attorney decided not to use his testimony as the previous medical testimony had not damaged his case, and he believed that his position was improved without the physician's testimony. In such cases, it is generally agreed that the doctor is entitled to similar compensation as if he had testified, although the fee may be adjusted according to the amount of time spent at the courthouse.

Last minute settlement or postponement of trial imposes a severe handicap in the practice of a medical specialist who performs frequent defense examinations. A significant number of these evaluations involve plaintiffs who have refused to settle their cases; the defendant insurance company often postpones the single examination to which it is entitled until a few weeks before trial date in the hope that an out-of-court settlement will make the examination unnecessary. If the plaintiff does not live in the area where the trial will be held, the defendant may not be able to have the evaluation until a day or two before trial, in order to have available a local medical witness with live testimony instead of the deposition of a physician from the plaintiff's locality. Because of these circumstances, the defendant expert testifies in a higher percentage of cases than a physician whose practice involves treatment of plaintiffs and few or no defendant evaluations. It becomes difficult for this expert to schedule surgery or office appointments as he is frequently placed on alert for trials. However, experience has demonstrated that approximately 75 per cent of the cases for which he is alerted never come to trial; they are either reset, postponed without a new trial date, or settled. The loss of time is increased for a trial in a town far removed from his office, as this necessitates cancellation of at least a half-day of his office time.

It is the usual practice of both plaintiffs and defendants to offer the doctor some compensation if his testimony is cancelled on the day set for trial. If the cancellation is made the previous day, the amount of compensation offered is minimal or none at all; usually any bill is met with strong resistance by either the plaintiff or defendant. The doctor is expected to absorb this loss as a cost of medico-legal practice. It is this type of occurrence which discourages many physicians from participating in medico-legal matters, as even twenty-four hours' notice is insufficient to rearrange a busy schedule of office appointments, surgery, and clinic obligations.

Attorneys should keep the doctor posted as the trial date nears, and check with him frequently while awaiting a court assignment and time. The trial does not always begin on the day scheduled, even in jurisdictions with a reputation for punctuality. There are many contingencies that arise in court proceedings such as need to hear criminal motions, interruptions to receive the verdict of a grand jury in a previous matter, or unexpected continuation of a preceding trial involving the plaintiff or defendant lawyer, making it impossible for him to begin a new judicial proceeding. Often the attorney himself is not responsible for the delay; in addition he does have other matters to consider besides the doctor—other witnesses, availability of his client, and other facets of his law practice. However, he still should remember the exceptional value of a busy doctor's time and make every effort to keep him informed of the exact time when his testimony will be required.

The attorney who calls or delivers a subpoena at 5:20 P.M. and states that he will need the doctor the following morning at 10:00 A.M., without any prior notice other than a letter several weeks before placing the doctor on a routine alert, is not realistic and cannot justifiably anticipate the doctor's full cooperation. It is the lawyer's obligation to keep his medical witnesses on notice; when there is no word from the attorney on the day before an alert, the doctor may assume that the case has either been settled or postponed.

In one such instance a busy specialist was called at 5:20 P.M. to testify the following day at 1:45 P.M. Two alerts for testimony in other cases on the same date had been cancelled the day before, and the doctor had then scheduled surgery at noon, followed by a full office schedule in his suburban clinic beginning at 2:00 P.M. In order to be present at trial as requested, it was necessary to cancel out one and a half hours of his appointments, two of which involved examinations on behalf of the same defendant for whom he was to testify. In addition, both of these cases were coming from out-of-state; long distance calls were made to reschedule them. The defendant attorney was reminded of the possibility that the patients might refuse to appear for the second appointment, as usually the defendant has only one chance to examine the plaintiff. The plaintiff could object to the second appointment if the doctor was responsible for the first cancellation.

In this case the doctor received a call at 11:00 A.M. and was advised the case in which he was to testify at 1:45 P.M. had been settled. It was apparent that the attorney had tried to settle the case the day before, and that was the reason why he had not notified the doctor until 5:20 P.M., after settlement negotiations had failed. Early that same morning the doctor had received still another call for defendant testimony in another case which had not been settled as anticipated. The doctor had been alerted several days before, but was given no further notice until a few hours before testimony was needed. He was asked to testify at the same hour he was scheduled to testify in the first case but in a far removed courthouse. The second attorney had been notified the doctor was unavailable, and he proceeded without his medical expert. Paradoxically, shortly after refusing the call, the doctor was informed by the first attorney that he had settled his case, but it was too late to be of help to the second attorney. This is an excellent example of the discouraging complexities of medico-legal practice.

Despite the gross inconvenience to the doctor imposed by a last minute request to testify, no compensation was paid to the doctor. Understandably, this led to an interruption in the physician's relations with this particular attorney. Such instances are very irritating but fortunately they do not occur very often. However, it is realistic to recognize that if the doctor has a large medico-legal practice, he is subject to frequent trial alerts, and occasionally many do fall on the same date and create a severe problem in his private medical practice.

FEES FOR DEFENDANT TESTIMONY AND EXAMINATIONS

Fees for defendant testimony vary with the amount of time involved for preparation for trial, travel time, and actual time the physician must be away from his medical practice. An important factor is whether the testimony is to be given at the convenience of the doctor or the convenience of the attorney. Usually the defendant attorney wishes his expert to appear after the plaintiff's doctor has testified, as this gives him an opportunity to rebut the other testimony, and also to develop additional points of evidence. If the order of testimony of the medical witnesses is reversed, the plaintiff's attorney is usually at a better advantage. In addition, if the plaintiff's physician has not yet testified, the defendant doctor may not be permitted to answer hypothetical questions based on anticipated testimony of the plaintiff's doctor. The two attorneys may agree in advance that such hypothetical questions will be permitted, but if such an agreement has not been made, then the defendant attorney is at a distinct disadvantage in rebutting testimony of the treating physician which was given after his witness has been excused.

Thus, if the defendant's expert must testify at a time resulting in additional loss of office appointments, then he should be permitted to charge a larger fee; if he must leave his office in the middle of his scheduled office hours, such as between 2 and 3 P.M., to give testimony and then return to his office, patient appointments will be missed, resulting in a greater loss of revenue and imposition upon his professional time. However, if he is able to testify immediately after the noon recess, the loss of time from his practice is less, as he is able to travel to court during the lunch period, and a lower fee is indicated.

A medical expert who develops into a recognized medico-legal authority with a talent for expert testimony and ability to withstand sharp cross-examination will soon find that his ability will not go unrecognized. His reputation is transmitted from one insurance company or defendant attorney to another, followed by frequent requests for defendant examinations and court appearances.

Although the doctor's expertise frequently results in defendant verdicts, or low plaintiff verdicts in cases of clear liability, thereby saving the defendant considerable sums of money, paradoxically such services are not always fully or promptly rewarded. Instead of receiving prompt payment of a reasonable charge for his professional services and time away from his office, he must often wait two to six months for payment, a situation necessitating irritating correspondence, phone calls, etc. because of the inefficiency or lackadaiscal attitude of the defendant's legal representative or insurance company. Most cases involve only one office visit, but the file must be kept open until payment is made, at which time it can be transferred to the inactive section. If the doctor sees a large number of cases for the defense, his active files soon become crowded, because many of these cases involve review of a thick portfolio of prior medical reports or depositions, to be used in preparation of his evaluation report and testimony.

The doctor should not be so committed to any insurance carrier or legal representative that they unjustifiably impose on his professional time without due compensation. Last minute cancellations of trial alerts and defendant examinations may result in considerable loss of appointment time or rescheduling of surgery, especially if the doctor has a large private practice. In most instances the physician should make a nominal charge for his lost time, but this of course is usually less than the customary fee for the service that was cancelled.

A significant percentage of plaintiff patients do not appear for their scheduled defendant examinations, having accepted the appointment against their desire; sometimes a court order is required to secure the examination, and even then some fail to appear. The loss of appointment time to a busy physician can be of considerable economic importance. Usually the doctor does not charge for this lost time, but if the patient fails to appear on a second occasion, the doctor should make a nominal charge for the lost appointment time (perhaps twenty-five dollars). Most insurance companies will absorb this cost or pass it on to the patient at settlement, but some do so reluctantly or even reject such a bill. This situation is paradoxical, as the services of a recognized medical expert, who has usually achieved that status because of his medico-legal talent and professional ability, are in demand. Such a physician will, in all probability, have developed a large medical practice (not related to medico-legal evaluations) which requires considerable professional time. He should be adequately compensated for any time devoted to the cause of the defendant who desires his services, even on occasion for unused time scheduled on the defendant's behalf. If the latter does not wish to be obligated to that extent financially, then he should seek the services of a physician who is not busy and has nothing better to do with his time. But the paradox is this: there is a good reason why that physician has so much free time—most likely he will not be able to provide the desired competence for the defendant's purpose.

FEES FOR DEPOSITIONS

In some instances, when the trial will be held in another city or the physician will be out of town on the trial date, a formal deposition may be requested instead of actual court testimony. If the physician is planning to be away at the time of the anticipated trial, he should promptly inform his attorney so that he may request a postponement of the trial or arrange for a deposition before the doctor leaves town. Although a deposition, which is later read by the attorney in open court and is not as strong evidence as live testimony, is taken under informal conditions, the usual legal procedures for testifying and cross-examination prevail. The deposition may be taken at the office of either the physician or attorney, at a mutually convenient time for all parties. The charge for deposition testimony depends upon the amount of time involved and resultant inconvenience to medical practice; generally the fee is less than that charged for a court appearance, frequently on a basis of fifty to seventy-five dollars per hour, or slightly higher in some communities.[29]

PRE-PAYMENT OF FEES FOR TESTIMONY

Some physicians request payment in advance before appearing in court for the plaintiff, especially if they cannot be assured of payment after trial because of lack of an assignment, poverty, questionable liability, unreliability of the claimant, etc. If this is the policy of the physician, he should make arrangements with the attorney for payment prior to trial, to avoid the distasteful conflicts which arise when he is subpoenaed to testify involuntarily. Once paid, however, he has entered into a contract to testify and must appear in court as agreed or face a possible lawsuit for breach of contract.

In some instances, especially when the physician's testimony is vital to a successful recovery of damages, the patient's attorney may advance the fee for his testimony if the plaintiff is financially unable to pay the doctor. Some attorneys may reject the physician's request for payment before going to the courthouse on the grounds that this is unethical legal practice. That is not the case, however, as the lawyer can ethically advance expenses subject to reimbursement (per Canon 42 of the Canons of Judicial Ethics, American Bar Association).[4]

TESTIMONY IN RESPONSE TO SUBPOENA WITHOUT FEE AGREEMENT

The physician may be subpoenaed to testify without mutual agreement, at which time he will be offered the ordinary witness fee required for the validity of the subpoena served upon him. In such instances he should promptly contact the attorney involved and try to agree upon a proper fee for expert testimony. If he is unsuccessful and must testify as an ordinary witness, usually he is not required to give an expert opinion but merely state the simple facts which came to his attention from examination and treatment of the patient. Under such circumstances the doctor would be wise to consult with his own attorney prior to appearing in court, as this is a controversial position which has not been finally resolved. Contradictory decisions of appellate courts are on record in several states as a result of a physician's refusal to give expert testimony without compensation. If he is asked to give an expert opinion during the trial, he may appeal to the judge for guidance, in order to avoid a citation for contempt of court, or ask for a recess to make arrangements for an expert witness fee before proceeding with further testimony. However, such incidents are rare, as the attorney who subpoenaes a doctor desires a favorable witness, and he usually has no wish to jeopardize his case for the relatively small sum of an expert witness fee.

ACCEPTANCE OF REDUCED FEES

The fee for testimony should be agreed upon in advance and be in no way dependent upon the outcome of trial or the size of the verdict. Any such understanding or agreement is unethical and cannot be condoned. However, the doctor may be faced with a decision to accept a reduced fee where the recovery has been minimal and insufficient to cover expenses. If the patient is destitute, there is no choice, but if the patient is working regularly and has other resources, the doctor should not accept a substantial reduction of his fee, particularly if his charges are reasonable and in accordance with the charges prevailing in that community.

In some instances he may make a settlement with the patient in order to obtain his reduced fee promptly, instead of partial payments over a prolonged period. In these circumstances it is customary for the plaintiff's attorney to obtain the doctor's consent before sending him a check for less than the full amount. The lawyer should inform him of the amount of the low recovery, and also any reduction in his legal fees, to help the doctor decide whether he will accept a reduced sum. The physician may request a copy of the settlement sheet for verification. Unless there is full disclosure the doctor should not accept a lower fee, as the lawyer may be transferring part of the doctor's bill to his client to influence him to accept a small settlement. A unilateral reduction of the fee by the attorney or patient without the consent of the physician is never acceptable and should not be tolerated. The doctor should also be sure the attorney is reducing his own fee in the same proportion as the physician's fee.

The above solution is no different than ordinary medical practice in which the doctor occasionally does not collect all of his fees; it is sometimes necessary to accept a reduced fee in order to obtain any payment at all. Some doctors have been known to raise their initial fees, anticipating a reduction at the time of settlement to their normal fee. This, however, represents an unethical practice; the physician should never pad his bill, but should charge a fair fee and then expect to receive that amount in full.

Another aspect, and one that is difficult to check, has been encountered with an occasional greedy, low-principled attorney who informs the doctor he must reduce his fee in order to obtain any recovery or settlement, but then proceeds to put his full bill on the settlement sheet handed to the client; inevitably this type of attorney pockets the difference and neither the doctor nor the patient realizes what has transpired. However, even though the doctor has a substantial medico-legal practice, the number of such cases is usually small. Should the physician become suspicious, he should contact the patient and request permission to inspect the settlement sheet.

The small financial loss from fee reductions is generally offset by a large volume of practice. It can be kept to a minimum by careful attention to, and shrewd interpretation of, requests for reductions in bills by both attorneys and patients. In many instances the patient is greedy and merely attempting to squeeze every penny out of the case regardless of the services rendered.

Most attorneys are reluctant to call the doctor to ask for a reduction of his fee, realizing that the bill was fair, represented actual services performed, and was not contingent in any way on the amount of the recovery. However, if his client insists on contacting the physician, it is preferable for the *attorney* to make the call; usually the physician will be contacted in a perfunctory manner, merely to satisfy the client's demands. If the doctor refuses to reduce his bill, the attorney may politely desist on his request, then inform the physician that he had made the call only at his patient's insistence. Most attorneys realize that the physician's future good will in other business contacts is more valuable than that of one individual client whom he may never see again.

6 QUALIFICATIONS

A PHYSICIAN IS AUTOMATICALLY DESIGNATED AS AN EXPERT WIT-
NESS IN ANY MEDICAL FIELD BECAUSE OF HIS EDUCATION, BUT THE
WEIGHT AND IMPACT OF HIS TESTIMONY IN A MEDICAL SPECIALTY IS
DIRECTLY DEPENDENT UPON HIS QUALIFICATIONS. THESE INCLUDE HIS
COLLEGE BACKGROUND, MEDICAL TRAINING, INTERNSHIPS, RESIDENCIES,
AND FELLOWSHIPS, ATTENDANCE AT SEMINARS AND SPECIAL TRAINING
PROGRAMS, CURRENT HOSPITAL APPOINTMENTS, TEACHING POSITIONS
AND AFFILIATION WITH MEDICAL SCHOOLS, CONSULTANT POSTS, AND
A SUMMARY OF PUBLISHED MEDICAL PAPERS AND SCIENTIFIC EXHIBITS.

The doctor who performs medico-legal examinations regularly
should prepare a memorandum of his qualifications for distribution to attorneys who request his services. This will facilitate the
presentation of his background and shorten his time in court, also
enhance his initial impression on the court and jury. He should
answer these questions briefly but fully, emphasizing the more
important current appointments. For example, it is not necessary
to give the dates and places of internships and residencies but
merely state "he had two years of surgical internship and three
years of surgical training." If there has been a pre-trial conference,
the attorney will have discussed this aspect of the testimony with
the doctor and he will be prepared for the questions.

The defendant attorney may rise to stipulate the qualifications of a well known medical expert without elaboration by the
witness. This may be accepted by the plaintiff attorney, especially
if the proceedings are nearing the noon recess or end of the day,
in order to complete the doctor's testimony without recalling him
to the witness stand and causing resultant impositions upon his
professional time. Usually, however, the plaintiff attorney wishes
to impress the jury with his witness' background and will ask the

doctor to summarize his qualifications; this should be done in a brief but thorough manner.

Judges who have had the medical expert in court on many occasions may interject their own comments when the defendant attorney admits the witness' qualifications, stating "the doctor is well known to this court and is qualified to give an expert opinion in his field." The wise plaintiff attorney realizes the judge wishes to expedite the judicial proceedings and does not ask further questions regarding the doctor's background, and proceeds with the testimony.

Usually there is little question regarding a doctor's credentials, especially when he is of good repute and well established in his field. However, in a recent trial proceeding, the defendant's witness observed that the plaintiff's attorney had made notes during the presentation of his qualifications as a medical expert, which is unusual. During the cross-examination, the lawyer questioned his background regarding his medical writings. He referred to a booklet widely distributed among doctors and attorneys entitled *Medico-Legal Examinations, Reports and Testimony.* This was an obvious attempt on the lawyer's part to depreciate the doctor's testimony by inferring he was a professional type of witness with medical research and writing as his principal occupation. The doctor pointed out that the booklet had been initially distributed at an annual convention of the American Academy of Orthopaedic Surgeons in 1966; the doctor had prepared a scientific exhibit on this subject, and the booklet was distributed to the orthopaedic surgeons who visited his booth, as clearly stated on the face of the booklet. When questioned regarding the nature of the pamphlet, the doctor testified that its purpose was to aid physicians in the preparation of medical reports, in order to facilitate the resolution of medico-legal cases under their care or in which they testified.

The final blow came when the presiding judge asked the doctor, as he was leaving the stand, if he would be kind enough to send him a few booklets for the use of himself and his fellow jurists. This certainly must have been impressive to the jury, and undoubtedly increased the weight of his evidence.

7 TESTIMONY

MEDICAL TESTIMONY IS ONLY OCCASIONALLY REQUIRED AFTER TREATMENT OR EXAMINATION OF PATIENTS INVOLVED IN ACCIDENTS, AS THE GREAT MAJORITY OF CASES ARE SETTLED OUT OF COURT. EVEN IN A BUSY MEDICO-LEGAL PRACTICE IT IS ESTIMATED THAT THE PHYSICIAN MUST APPEAR IN COURT IN LESS THAN FIVE PER CENT OF HIS PLAINTIFF CASES. DEFENDANT EXAMINATIONS RESULT IN A HIGHER INCIDENCE OF COURT TESTIMONY, AS OFTEN THESE CASES ARE REFERRED FOR EVALUATION AFTER SETTLEMENT NEGOTIATIONS FAIL AND TRIAL APPEARS INEVITABLE.

IMPORTANCE AND VALUE

Although many physicians are apprehensive of appearing before a jury or court, the experience does not necessarily have to be unpleasant or lengthy if the physician is well informed and cooperates with the attorney who summons him to court.

A properly prepared physician often finds his courtroom experience educational and not as traumatic as he had anticipated. However, his introduction to the legal process may be unpleasant if he is irritated by an aggressive plaintiff or defendant attorney. If he is not familiar with the procedural rules, he may be at a loss to understand what is required of him; as a result a communications breakdown occurs which prevents an intelligent discussion and presentation of medical issues, usually to the detriment of his patient, the plaintiff. The doctor's appearance in court does not have to be uncomfortable or traumatic if he is briefed beforehand regarding the rules of evidence which he must follow when testifying. If he is better informed about medico-legal procedures, his inevitable courtroom appearance will be more meaningful, uncomplicated, and of briefer duration.

There are few doctors who enjoy giving testimony, or are neutral about requests to appear as a witness in court. The few who do welcome the remuneration and attention resulting from court testimony are often identified as professional witnesses, either as a defendant's medical expert who usually favors the insurance company, or as a plaintiff's witness who will usually give a positive causal relationship between an accident and the alleged resultant disability. The reluctance of most physicians to participate in medico-legal matters results in a low percentage of doctors representing the entire profession in court; usually this small number does not portray a representative cross section of physicians.[31]

Although divisions of medical opinion will continue, more willingness by physicians to take the witness stand would assure a higher quality of medical testimony. It would also involve physicians who are actually treating the patient, in the presentation of testimony, rather than special medico-legal consultants who examine the patient for the specific purpose of testifying. Usually the actively involved treating physician is somewhat reluctant to be a witness in the case. Although he could be summoned to court for this purpose, subpoenaed witnesses have often been found to give undesirable testimony, and attorneys try to avoid that situation.

The reluctance of physicians to become medical witnesses arises from many factors, principally the pressures of their private practice, which is disrupted all too often by unforeseen delays during the courtroom process—such as early adjournment, bench conferences, chamber conferences, research of points of law, and so on. Other restraints are a fear of merciless cross-examination, harassment, even the recall and public display of unfavorable previous episodes in the doctor's personal life or professional career. In addition there are the personal reactions of physicians to the trial technique, such as the challenging of his opinions, the necessity to adhere to courtroom principles, the inability to speak freely without interruption, or to deliver a lecture based on his opinions, the relatively small fee of the physician for crucial testimony as compared to the often enormous contingent fee the attorney receives, and of course there is professional pride. For most physicians, the courtroom tribunal offers an unfamiliar setting, an untried situation. . . . The medical witness who appears in court only occasionally, is ill at ease and often unhappy to be forced to participate in the judicial proceedings.

MANNER AND TIME OF TESTIMONY

The doctor should report to the courtroom fully prepared to testify. He should have reviewed his records, placed them in chronological order, and be fully cognizant of the contents of his file. This advance preparation will permit him to refer to his notes in an efficient manner without delaying his testimony. Nothing is more irritating to the judge and jury than to wait patiently while the witness fumbles through his briefcase or file in search of records needed to answer an attorney's question. The physician's testimony is enhanced by an efficient and prompt manner when he must refer to his notes and medical records. Extraneous material, such as letters of referral, for which he will have no need in his testimony, should be temporarily extracted from the file before he takes the stand.

The time for the physician's appearance should be pre-arranged with the attorney requesting his services, in order to conserve the physician's professional time. Usually the physician can be placed on telephone call or advised to appear at a specific time, such as immediately after the luncheon recess. Both the examining and treating physicians are often served a subpoena for legal purposes to insure their appearance and testimony and to protect their client; in these instances the attorney should alert the physician that a subpoena will be served upon him, but that he should await a telephone call before appearing in court.

If the subpoena is received without prior notice, the doctor should phone the attorney and arrange a set time for his testimony, instead of reporting when the court convenes as directed by the subpoena. The physician should realize the legal necessity of the subpoena and not resent it; without it, the attorney is defenseless before the judge if the medical expert suddenly decides not to appear or is unavoidably detained. The validity of the subpoena depends on the jurisdiction of the court; if it is a federal court it has a wider area of effectiveness than a municipal or county court, and the subpoena is valid for a considerable distance from the doctor's office. If he has any doubts, the subpoenaed physician may phone the clerk of the court for information and guidance.

There are few circumstances which will permit the doctor to be excused from compliance with a valid subpoena. If he has surgery scheduled at a time in conflict with his subpoenaed court appearance, he may be temporarily excused by arrangement with the attorney who issued the subpoena or with the presiding judge, but this may not necessarily hold; in fact, he may be forced to cancel the operation if ordered to comply with the subpoena as issued. If he has advance knowledge of the trial, the physician may be excused from testifying, or may ask postponement of the trial in order to attend a medical convention or seminar, especially if he has already registered or made reservations to attend that meeting. This has been supported by court decisions, such as the ruling of the New York Superior Court to the effect that physicians' attendance at a medical meeting justified delay of a trial and the granting of a new trial date (*Strakoski* vs *Bullock*, 316, N.Y.S. 2d, 834—N.Y. Superior Court, App. Div., Nov 5, 1970).[36]

The witness should make his appearance on time or preferably a few minutes earlier, in the event the court proceedings have advanced further than anticipated. Usually the attorney has notified the judge of the time scheduled for the doctor's appearance, and it is essential that the latter be in court at the appointed time. Most judges, but not all, will give the physician some preference in taking the stand, sometimes interrupting the testimony of a lay witness to permit the physician to testify without delay. This is especially true when the doctor has established a reputation before that jurist for promptness and cooperation. In some instances a short recess may be declared while the court is awaiting the doctor's arrival, instead of putting another witness on the stand, to accommodate the physician. Should he enter the courtroom more than a few minutes late under those circumstances, it would be appropriate to apologize to the court and explain the reason for his delay—surgery, emergency case, or other obligation. However, the physician must understand that the attorney has problems related to the successful presentation of his case, and may not wish to interrupt a witness' testimony to accommodate the physician's schedule.

Thus it is not always possible for the doctor's testimony to be taken immediately upon his appearance at the trial. Not infrequently, he is asked to have a seat outside and wait for the witness on the stand to complete his testimony. The waiting doctor may be impressed with the aura of importance and seriousness which permeates the courtroom halls and waiting rooms. Clerks and bailiffs stroll past without greeting, intent upon their impartial role in the judicial proceedings. Other witnesses are impatiently waiting, some held over from the day before; they resent the preference given to the medical witness who is called to the stand shortly after he makes his presence known. While sitting outside the courtroom, the medical witness should use this time to again review his records, thoroughly familiarize himself with the details in all medical reports, and relax until he is called to the stand. Under no circumstances should he discuss the case in any regard with any other witness. His time on the witness stand will be materially shortened and his impression upon the jury more favorable if he does not have to rattle through his folder in answer to each question, but instead is able to respond promptly and decisively without reference to his notes.

Occasionally there may be a directed verdict or a court recess and settlement before the physician's testimony is given: this could result from incontrovertible testimony rejecting liability or from the failure of the plaintiff to present sufficient evidence to establish his case. This outcome should be looked upon as an unavoidable result of the judicial process, and the physician should accept the interruption to his professional routine without resentment. However, he should make a charge for the time lost from his practice and care of patients.

Most medico-legal experts agree that the medical witness

should dress in a conservative, dignified manner, avoiding loud, flamboyant *way-out* clothes. Obviously, he should always wear a tie and jacket, even though he may be testifying in a rural county court. Almost all jurors are properly attired, and will probably resent the appearance of a witness who does not show the respect due the court in his manner of dress.

On arrival at the courthouse the doctor should immediately notify the attorney of his presence by sending him word by way of the bailiff, or else by briefly entering the courtroom and gaining the attention of either the bailiff or the attorney, then waiting outside (usually there is a rule on witnesses and he cannot wait inside the courtroom). The bailiff will lead him to the stand when the court is ready for his testimony. The witness should pause before taking a seat and turn towards the clerk of the court, who will then place him under oath. After nodding a greeting to the judge and being seated, he should arrange his notes in front of him and face the attorney who will be questioning him. At this point his composure and mannerisms are very important in their effect on the jury. His attitude should be that of a neutral witness. He should address his remarks to the jury but should not try to influence them with a beaming, supercilious smile. The doctor should make his remarks in an audible even voice, avoiding dramatic emphasis in his replies unless forced to do so by the cross-examiner. Under no circumstances should he assume the posture of an infallible expert and address his remarks to the court with a condescending or patronizing air. The jurors recognize that the doctor has specialized technical knowledge, but they will resent any witness who *talks down* to them.

He should talk to the jury in a calm, modest manner, with authority, but with care not to pontificate or appear smug (Figure 18). He should use a normal tone of voice in the manner of an individual who knows his subject, but without the aura of ultimate authority. The physician should answer questions fully, but should not elaborate, as usually this leads to further inquiry he himself precipitated by bringing up new subjects. Lengthy replies will only lead to objections by the opposition attorney and characterization of the witness as an advocate. Again, his discussions should be directed toward the jury, explaining any unavoidable medical terms and reducing technical terminology to a minimum; he should constantly remember he is addressing a lay audience.

The physician on the stand should remember that the opposing attorney has intensely reviewed the case and is probably familiar with its medical aspects. The physician has nothing to fear if he knows his subject, as an attorney cannot equal his medical knowledge after only a brief period of study; however, it is surprising how well informed an astute, interested lawyer can be if he thoroughly prepares and researches the subject before the trial. The physician must be equally prepared by a pre-trial review of the anatomy and clinical considerations involved in that particular case.

When asked to answer *yes* or *no*, he should do so if possible, but if a more complete answer is indicated, he should qualify his answer or indicate to the court he is unable to give an informative answer by the simple word *yes* or *no*, and that an explanation is required in more detail. Usually the court will permit the witness to give a proper reply.

The physician should never exaggerate concerning either his own qualifications or the extent of the findings in his examination. To do so is to lead to exposure and resultant embarrassment. A physician who is well prepared and reports to the courtroom with adequate records has nothing to fear if he tells the truth without exaggeration or embellishment. He should be careful not to appear as an advocate for the party calling him to the stand. He should not overtly signal to his counsel while on the witness stand, or manifest, by facial expression or words, a feeling of victory in his responses to challenging questions from the opposing attorney. When leaving the court, he may nod to the judge as a *thank-you* gesture for dismissing him, but he should not speak or gesture to the attorney for whom he testified, nor should he sit beside and counsel his attorney during the remainder of the trial, as the jury will then recognize his partisanship. The physician should "let the chips fall where they may," and, if there is a disability, he should state it clearly; if, on the other hand, he believes there is exaggeration or lack of objectivity in the complaints, he should also state that in his testimony. His principal objective is to enlighten the jury, not to impress or prejudice them.

The physician should remember that testimony in a courtroom is before an audience of considerable experience, as trial judges are accustomed to medical evaluation. Judge Stevens Fargo of Los Angeles has noted that juries represent a combined total of four hundred to five hundred years of human experience. He further observed, "While juries are prepared to receive the doctor's evidence on a favorable basis, due to the esteem we all have for the profession, they are seldom bamboozled and to my observation are not receptive to testimony of a doctor who becomes an advocate."[8]

Testimony given in response to cross-examination merits separate discussion, as the questions are then being directed by a hostile attorney instead of the attorney who requested the doctor's appearance. Suggestions for responses to cross-examination are given in a separate section (pp. 279–314).

SUBPOENA AS ORDINARY WITNESS

The doctor will undoubtedly be irritated if he is subpoenaed as an ordinary witness instead of as an expert, receiving a fee of only a few dollars instead of an amount consistent with his earning power and the time expended. However, with proper preparation and some arrangements with the counsel calling him to court, the doctor will, in most instances, be compensated as an expert and will not be forced to accept the subpoena fee. A Pennsylvania decision stated that "the litigant has no more right to compel a citizen to give up the product of his brain than he has to compel the giving up of material things." However, several jurisdictions do compel the doctor to answer without compensation as an expert when he has been subpoenaed to court without arrangements for an expert witness fee. At the same time most attorneys realize that considerable damage can be done to their case in such a situation as the witness is often hostile and uncooperative under the circumstances. If the judge directs the witness to answer a question, he cannot refuse to reply; otherwise he will

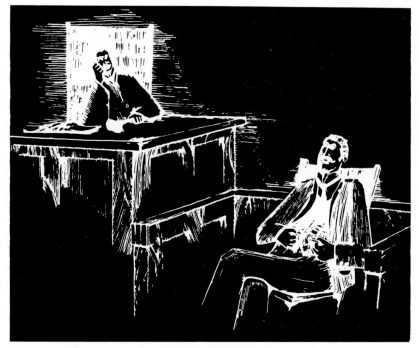

FIGURE 18. DON'T PONTIFICATE—GIVE TESTIMONY,
NOT A LECTURE.

be subject to a citation for contempt of court. However, the
content of his reply is at his discretion—"I have no opinion," may
be a desirable answer in this situation. If he has no opinion, he
cannot be questioned on that point any further.

The type of testimony which the doctor must give in response
to a subpoena, when he appears involuntarily and without previous agreement wih the attorney regarding his fees, constitutes
a problem which often perplexes the physician witness. Usually
he is required to testify only as to facts, as contrasted to opinions
resulting from medical judgment. Ordinary facts include history,
objective physical findings, and treatment. Diagnosis and prognosis are based on interpretation of the facts; usually the judge
will sustain the refusal of a medical witness to answer questions
related to these phases of his examination when he is not being
compensated as an expert. This situation often results in a recalci-

trant witness of little value to the attorney who calls him, but if the subpoenaed doctor is a treating physician who is not familiar with his legal rights, a clever attorney may extract from him considerable information of value to his case. Generally it is agreed that the best witness is one for whom fair compensation has been arranged in advance and who reports to court voluntarily.

In a recent case, which had been postponed three times and had been pending for six years, the case finally came to trial at a time when the treating physician was unexpectedly out of the city. As a result, the plaintiff's attorney had no medical evidence to support his client's claim of injury which she made during her testimony. At the noon recess he subpoenaed the defendant orthopaedic expert, who had examined the husband and wife one year previously and submitted reports to the defendant attorney, to appear in court at 2:00 P.M. the same day. Although the reports were generally unfavorable to the plaintiff's case, they did disclose certain injuries. Apparently it was the plaintiff attorney's hope to at least establish some type of injury, even though most of the report would be harmful to his case.

The defendant attorney had not phoned the doctor or notified him that the case was in progress, although he had sent him a letter two weeks previously alerting him to the need for testimony on that day. The doctor had assumed the case had been settled and the defendant attorney had forgotten to notify his medical witness (this happens much too often!). The defendant orthopaedist was served with a subpoena from the plaintiff attorney without the witness fee. He pointed out to the process server (who unfortunately happened to be the attorney's law clerk) that without a fee this was not a valid subpoena (an obvious mistake); a few minutes later the process server returned with the standard fee, which then obligated the physician to be on telephone call for testimony that day.

The doctor was forced to cancel a tennis match on a beautiful summer day as he was called to court in the early afternoon. After being sworn in, the plaintiff's attorney attempted to qualify the doctor as an expert but the witness responded that he was testifying as an ordinary witness and was not in court as a physician or as an expert (a physician is a *de facto* expert by his very training and professional qualifications). The judge immediately commented, "Apparently, the doctor has been very well instructed; he is absolutely correct." The defense attorney then attempted by various methods to get into evidence the report submitted by the doctor. When shown the report, he testified to the fact that it was his report, but when questioned about the content, he again refused to answer on the grounds that this was knowledge obtained as an expert. The judge concurred in the doctor's statement, and advised the attorney that he could not question him as an expert as he had not been so qualified.

At this point the judge turned to the jury members and explained the situation to them; he advised them that the doctor was not being hostile but was entitled to a fee commensurate with his expertise and time lost from the office. He advised the jury that it is customary for an expert doctor to charge a substantial fee as an expert witness, but in this case he was being paid $20.80 as an ordinary witness.

As a last resort the plaintiff attorney obviously tried to cause a mistrial, in order to create another opportunity for him to obtain medical testimony when his own doctor had returned from vacation. He asked the doctor whether the defendant sitting at the table had paid his bill, apparently hoping that the doctor would answer that it was paid by his insurance company; however, the doctor recognized the trap and answered only that his bill was paid by the defendant's representative. As a last resort, the plaintiff attorney requested the doctor to state what his fee would be as an expert witness, but the judge overruled him and refused to permit an answer, stating that this was not pertinent at this point.

After a few more frustrating questions, the plaintiff attorney realized that he could not obtain any information and the witness was excused. The defendant attorney declined to cross-examine his witness, realizing that he could not improve the benefits already derived from the direct examination. The result was a minimal verdict in favor of the plaintiff sufficient to pay only property damage and medical bills—although the attorney took one-third of this!

The above illustration demonstrates the necessity for cooperation between physician and attorney, especially when the doctor is placed in a difficult position and called upon to testify under adverse circumstances. If the doctor is inexperienced in court procedures, he should consult his own attorney for information and guidance before reporting to the courthouse. In this particular case, the orthopaedist had a great deal of court experience and realized his rights and privileges. When in doubt while on the witness stand, the physician may ask the court's permission to refuse to answer certain questions, stating his reply would constitute an opinion, and he understands that, as an ordinary witness, he is obligated to testify only with regard to facts. A diagnosis is an opinion and does not have to be offered. However, if the judge directs the witness to answer the question, he must do so or risk a citation for contempt of court (as previously mentioned). In this case, the plaintiff attorney also attempted to obtain the history from the doctor, but the judge overruled this as "hearsay evidence."

A strange aftermath of this case was a letter received from the plaintiff's attorney three days after the trial, advising the doctor that the minimal check of $20.80 for an ordinary witness was being stopped for payment:

Dear Dr. Brown:

With reference to the subpoena delivered to you on October 25, 1970, please be advised that your services as a witness are no longer required on November 25, 1970, and therefore payment has been stopped on our check no. 4379, which was also delivered to you.

Thank you for your cooperation, and please accept our apologies for any scheduling inconvenience this matter may have caused you.

With regards,
Fred Austin, Esq.

The basis for the stop payment was a typographical error on the subpoena that had been delivered on October 25, 1970 at

1:00 P.M., requiring testimony that same afternoon; *November* had been typed instead of *October*. The error had been mentioned by the plaintiff's attorney as he ceased his questioning of the witness; his law clerk brought this to his attention to indicate that the doctor had appeared voluntarily and not in response to a subpoena (wrong date), and thus could testify as an expert. However, the judge ruled that this error had no bearing on the doctor's refusal to testify as an expert witness under the circumstances. Inasmuch as the trial has been concluded on October 25, it was perfectly obvious that the plaintiff's attorney was using the typographical error as a method of vengeance against the subpoenaed physician, despite his polite language. Although the physician could have obtained a favorable judgment for twenty dollars and eighty cents by a civil suit, it was obviously not worth the time and expense involved, a fact the plaintiff's attorney undoubtedly understood.

However, he apparently did not anticipate that the doctor would bring the matter to the attention of the local Bar Association and its grievance committee, in view of the attorney's unprofessional ethics and behavior. This complaint led to prompt payment and conclusion of this incident, but the attorney still had several plaintiff cases pending with this orthopaedist. As is to be expected, he alienated that physician from further professional relationships with his office. Another unusual facet was that the orthopaedist had successfully treated the same plaintiff attorney for a back injury only a short time before the incident, and also had treated several clients referred by that attorney. The cases were still pending at the time of the above incident; obviously the attorney could not anticipate any cooperation from the doctor if these cases should come to trial. Here then would be a strong factor in forcing an unfavorable settlement, bound to result in a reduction in the attorney's contingent fee; this reduction, by the way, would amount to far more than the $20.80 he attempted to save by stopping his check for the subpoena. The old adage of cutting off your nose to spite your face certainly appears to be pertinent to this experience.

Another example of a request for expert testimony without compensation appears in the following incident in the course of which an orthopaedist had examined a patient in a Virginia hospital. The plaintiff attempted to serve a subpoena upon the doctor to take his deposition a week before the trial in a town fifty-five miles away, even though he had been furnished with the doctor's medical report. The plaintiff was unsuccessful in this attempt as the doctor had no office in Virginia and, when alerted to the subpoena, remained out of the state until the trial. The plaintiff's attorney made no tender of transportation expenses or any witness fee. The doctor later learned that if he had been served with the subpoena, he would have been required to appear, as the laws of Virginia do not require a tender of witness fees or expense money as they do in Washington, D.C. Of course, if the doctor had appeared, he could have refused to allow himself to be qualified as an expert unless the attorney paid him in advance for his expenses and testimony. However, he would have had the annoyance of 110 miles of travel and cancellation of his office hours without compensation.

In this case the patient had been injured in two automobile accidents two years apart, and had received treatment after each accident. When his case came to trial for the second accident, neither the general practitioner nor the orthopaedic or neurosurgical consultants were able to definitely link the patient's complaints solely with the second accident; they stated they could not clearly differentiate the complaints from those arising from the preceding accident of two years before. One of the doctors stated that he had no idea that the man had been in a second accident. It was clearly evident throughout the claimant's testimony that he was either exaggerating or grossly misrepresenting the facts, even contradicting the records of his family doctor. In this case justice prevailed and the jury rendered a defendant's verdict. The plaintiff's attorney was saddled with court expenses and received no fee as he was on the usual contingency basis. Perhaps this was his reward for having tried to subpoena the doctor to a distant town without financial compensation!

SIGNIFICANCE OF VOLUNTARY AGREEMENT TO TESTIFY

When the doctor has voluntarily agreed to testify without a subpoena, it has been established that he has made a contract and is legally liable to appear in court at the designated time. If an agreement has been made regarding the fee, and especially if the fee has been paid in advance, his failure to appear makes him liable for legal action. The doctor must realize that once he has made an agreement to testify, he is legally obligated to appear in court. If a medical emergency occurs to interfere with his court appearance, he should notify the court immediately, then abide by the decision of the judge whether or not he is excused; otherwise he is liable to suit, as noted in the ruling of *Battista* vs *Bellino:*

"PHYSICIANS AND SURGEONS"—Action for Breach of

Contract to Testify

The Superior Court of New Jersey, Appellate Division, has upheld a complaint stating a cause of action against plaintiff's treating physician for breach of contract to testify in her personal injury action which she alleged had resulted in a smaller recovery than would have been achieved had the doctor been present to testify at the proper time. The allegations were that the doctor, though he had been paid to do so, had failed to appear, that the plaintiff had been required to rest, and that the doctor had appeared only the next day when it was too late to give evidence (*Battista* vs *Bellino*, March 1, 1971, 274A–2d595, Opinion by Judge Mountain).

The facts in this case were as follows: a woman was injured in an automobile accident, following which she and her husband brought suit against the driver of the other car involved in the collision. The counsel for the injured woman arranged for the treating physician to testify as to her injuries. Although he was paid a fee of two hundred dollars in advance, he did not appear at the trial and could not be located on that day. When the counsel and physician appeared in court the following morning, the trial judge did not permit the physician to testify because the opposing medical witnesses had been released the previous afternoon, and the defendant would not be able to counter the physician's testimony. The jury awarded the woman 2,500 dollars.

The couple brought action against the physician, claiming that he had entered into a contract to testify on their behalf and that they were injured as a result.[4,36]

CONTEMPT OF COURT FOR FAILURE TO COMPLY WITH SUBPOENA

The preceding case is an illustration of the violation of a voluntary agreement without a subpoena. However, if the doctor has been properly served with a valid subpoena, he is under a stronger obligation to comply, unless he is properly excused. Many subpoenae have a notation at the bottom, that the doctor may phone the attorney issuing the summons and be placed on telephone call, in order to minimize loss of time from his practice. If this can be satisfactorily arranged, the doctor may appear according to such an arrangement. Otherwise he is legally obligated to appear in court at the time and place designated on the subpoena.

A recent article in *Medical Tribune* reports that a Charlotte, North Carolina physician was fined one hundred dollars on each of two contempt-of-court charges for failure to answer a subpoena to testify in a personal injury case. When the doctor failed to appear, the judge ordered the physician brought in by the sheriff. The physician and sheriff arrived after court had recessed and the physician was told to report back at 9:30 A.M. the next day. The doctor did report back the following morning, but at 10:00 A.M. instead of 9:30 A.M. He was levied a fine of one hundred dollars for contempt of court on the first violation, and he was ordered to reappear in court the following week for his late appearance in court on the second day. At the second hearing he was found guilty and fined an additional one hundred dollars. The judge explained that the physician had kept the jury waiting one hour the first day, and on the second day the trial was forced to continue without his testimony. The doctor's explanation that he "was late because he could not find the necessary records" was unacceptable and rejected.

All of this unpleasantness could have been avoided by a simple phone call to the court to make arrangements for his testimony. The details of the case were not cited, but it is suspected that there were prior difficulties between the client, attorney, and physician due to the doctor's lack of cooperation or interest in the legal proceedings.

PRE–TRIAL CONFERENCE WITH ATTORNEY

In most instances a pre-trial conference between physician and attorney will be helpful in securing information and guidance for both parties. The attorney may stress the evidence he desires to be emphasized in court and advise the physician how to avoid argumentative or controversial points; this will better prepare the physician to testify and respond to cross-examination. Sometimes the conference may result in a settlement of the litigation, by clarifying the medical issues for the attorney. This is especially true if there is little difference in the medical opinions of both the plaintiff and defendant physicians, or if the lawyer's preconceived estimate of the patient's injuries and disability was grossly inaccurate; after hearing the doctor's proposed testimony, the attorney may leave the conference with a firm determination to settle the case as best he can.

It is recommended that this conference be scheduled at the end of the day, when there will be no interruptions from phone calls or patients. Skeletal diagrams or plastic skeletons, posters, and x-rays pertaining to the case are valuable visual aids in the instruction and preparation of the attorney. Residual disability should be clearly defined without hesitation and with no attempt to minimize or exaggerate, as there is no advantage for an attorney to have an incorrect perspective of his case when he faces his antagonist in court. The other attorney has undoubtedly had medical conferences also to help prepare his case, and is probably aware of the actual facts.

TESTIMONY REGARDING MALINGERING

At times the physician testifying for the defense may be asked his opinion as to whether or not the plaintiff is malingering.

Wherever possible, the doctor should avoid using that term, even though he may be correct in doing so, as the jurors may be adversely affected by his opinion. Some jurors are skeptical of defendant experts, especially if they are so extreme that they label the plaintiff as a *liar,* and the plaintiff is a sweet attractive lady!

The physician's answer should review his findings, stating that the objective clinical and x-ray examination did not substantiate the patient's continuing complaints, that the symptoms were completely inconsistent with the negative findings, and that as a result he believed the complaints were grossly exaggerated. An opinion regarding malingering would involve the questions of psychiatric review, psycho-social background, mental attitudes, and other factors; these questions are beyond the province of a physician who was asked to perform only a medical examination, not an evaluation of character and morals. The court and jury, who will have heard all the testimony in the case (not just the medical) and are aware of other instances of probable fabrication and inconsistencies, are in a better position to evaluate character than the examining physician.

Therefore, the doctor should limit his statement by saying that he was unable to discover any objective findings to explain the continued complaints, but that he does not believe he is in a position to pass judgment upon the plaintiff's character; the doctor would thereupon suggest that he is unable to give an opinion whether the patient is malingering. He may add that he believes the court, who has heard all the evidence, is in a better position to make such a conclusion. If you do indicate the patient is probably a "malingerer" and the jury disagrees with your characterization of the claimant, the remainder of your testimony may be discredited.

INTRODUCTION OF SURPRISE MEDICAL EVIDENCE

A case recently came to trial in which the primary complaints referred to the cervical spine, although the patient (a middle-aged female) did have some complaints in the lower back. The patient had been examined sixteen months after the accident by a defendant physician, at which time he found no evidence of any residuals of injury to her neck or back. The objective clinical findings and x-rays were normal for both the cervical and lumbar spines. He did observe considerable nervous tension, most likely related to a functional disorder. She still complained of some discomfort in the lumbar spine, which was believed to be non-anatomical in origin; there was no evidence of muscle spasm and all clinical tests were negative at that time.

During the plaintiff's presentation of her case the treating physician testified that surgery would probably be indicated for her lower back. This was the first time such a claim had been made, and there had been no pre-trial indication of this unexpected development. The judge ruled there had been a mistrial. Subsequently, the plaintiff's attorney requested the physician to re-examine his patient and submit a more detailed report which would sustain the statements made at trial, as in his pre-trial reports surgery had never been mentioned.

It was quite evident that this surprise testimony was a gross exaggeration and misrepresentation which exceeded the clinical findings; it was also obvious that the physician was taking an advocate position. His pre-trial reports were concerned mostly with her cervical complaints, not her low back. In his later report, given after the mistrial, he not only indicated the anticipated surgery, but he discussed all possible complications of such surgery—post-operative infection, leading to draining sinuses, then more surgery, followed by amyloid infiltration of the liver and kidneys, etc. He did omit the possibility of cardiac arrest and pulmonary embolism!

USE OF EXHIBITS

It is sometimes difficult for the witness to present testimony on scientific or medical subjects in a manner which will be clearly understood by the court and jury. His language must be non-technical and should, as much as possible, be simplified; when unfamiliar terms are used, they should be explained. In many instances, an exhibit of such items as a technical apparatus, photographs, illustrations, or a partial skeleton, will more clearly indicate to the court and jury the points which the doctor wishes to emphasize. Blackboard sketches made during the testimony are also useful, but should only be used by physicians who have some skill at drawing. A sloppy demonstration is worse than no demonstration at all.

Technical apparatus, such as a Jamar grip tester or a Cervigon apparatus, may be quite helpful in demonstrating how the physician measures range of motion, grip testing, and so on. If it is not practical to bring in the actual apparatus, he may bring the photograph or illustration of the apparatus which is often supplied in the manufacturer's instructions accompanying the equipment. Partial skeletons made of plastic are now available for almost all parts of the body and are very useful in demonstrating anatomical parts or areas of injury. Large diagrams of skeletons, muscles, nerves, and blood vessels are also available commercially for demonstration purposes.

The doctor must decide in advance to what extent he wishes to participate in the case being tried. It is the author's opinion that he should use whatever technical means are necessary to illustrate his medical testimony, but that he should not become an advocate, and should restrain himself in the use of such exhibits and illustrations. He should refrain from becoming a professional witness who tries to influence the jury in favor of the party for whom he is testifying, but should present the facts in a fair, thorough, and impartial manner. Some physicians lean over the jury box, beam at the jurors and make an obvious attempt to solicit the sympathy and support of the jury members by their manner of speech and address. It is the author's opinion that this is beyond the province of an impartial medical witness. He should have no interest in the outcome, and his fees are the same—win, lose or draw!

Attorney Jack E. Horsley, in a recent article, warns physicians that they should prepare for testimony by carefully reviewing the illustrations and exhibits with their attorney; they should also be sure that the equipment is in good mechanical working condition. It obviously would be embarrassing to have an exhibit fail in an open courtroom demonstration; this would certainly detract from the testimony being given.[22]

MEDICAL RECORDS IN THE COURTROOM

The doctor should bring all pertinent medical records to court *after* he has carefully reviewed these records and removed any personal or embarrassing correspondence (from the attorney or insurance company). This would include notations or correspondence regarding the doctor's fee for the examination and testimony, memoranda to the doctor informing him the carrier has knowledge of prior unreported accidents and claims, request to take a detailed history of previous injuries, a strongly worded opinion of the insurance adjuster or defendant attorney to the effect that he believes the patient is faking, notes informing the examining physician that the accident caused very minor property damage and that the patient had told the officer on the scene that she was not hurt, or similar correspondence.

The physician should also remember, when making notations in his medical records, that these records are often intensely reviewed by the opposing attorney in open court, and that they may lead to harassing questions. Only too often a physician hurries to court with a folder which he has not reviewed and which contains letters from the attorney or insurance company, or personal notes which were better left in the office. Had the doctor studied and sorted the contents of the folder he would have spared himself considerable embarrassment from questions put to him in court.

A statement of charges should be brought to court, preferably itemized, as a simple lump sum bill is often not acceptable and may invite challenges regarding its fairness.

X-RAYS—BRING THEM TO COURT!

The doctor should always take the patient's x-rays with him when reporting to court for testimony, even though they are completely normal or "negative." Prior evidence may have been given necessitating the use of these films as evidence, and they should be available. If the films are left in the office, it is impossible or very difficult to obtain them in time to utilize them while the doctor is on the witness stand.

The value of negative films is well exemplified by the following incident. The author was called to testify as an expert in a low back injury case in nearby Virginia. From previous medical reports of the treating physician and a defendant examination, it appeared to be a routine low back strain with no allegation of other injury. However, the plaintiff's doctor gave surprise testimony (just ahead of the defendant's medical witness) that the patient had a herniated lumbar disc syndrome, based solely on progressive narrowing of the lumbosacral interspace as demonstrated in two sets of x-ray films taken in his office one year apart. He found no symptoms or objective signs of a disc or other evidence that would suggest disc pathology, other than the apparent narrowing on the second set of x-ray films.

The patient had been examined by the defendant's physician just one week prior to trial; lumbosacral x-rays were made in the same week that the treating physician had taken his second set of films. The roentgenograms made by the defendant's physician showed an intact intervertebral disc space with no evidence of any narrowing. The films made by the plaintiff's physician a few days later showed some apparent narrowing in the posterior half of the interspace, but these films were taken off-center and at a slight angle. In his testimony the defendant physician pointed out the difference in x-ray technique between the films of 1970 and 1971, and also stated that his own films had shown findings comparable to those made in 1970. However, he did not have the films with him in court (he had inadvertently left them in his office) and was unable to demonstrate them. He indicated the varying techniques in the two sets of films, and also the lack of any sclerosis, spurring or other degenerative changes which would be consistent with progressive narrowing and degeneration of the lumbosacral disc. However, had he brought his own films to court, there would have been dramatic corroboration of his testimony on this point, as his recent films were identical to those made one year earlier by the plaintiff's doctor.

The patient received a verdict of five thousand dollars in a case in which there was full liability and in which there was some residual of a low back strain; it is quite possible that this verdict would have been diminished had the defendant's x-rays been available for demonstration in court. Ironically, the defendant attorney had phoned the doctor at the lunch recess and asked him to hurry to court, but forgot to request him to bring his x-rays, even though the plaintiff's expert had already testified and inserted the disc problem into the proceedings. Thus it is good policy to be prepared to give the best possible testimony by bringing all x-rays to court.

REVIEW OF PRIOR X-RAYS

The testifying physician should review all x-rays prior to trial. Whenever possible, previous x-rays should be secured to compare to present ones, in order to determine whether the accident has caused traumatic aggravation of any pre-existing defects such as arthritis or a degenerative disc syndrome, or whether there was any reversal or alteration of spinal curves immediately after the accident. Usually such x-rays can be secured by a direct phone call to the physician or radiologist where they were made, but occasionally an overprotective plaintiff or defendant attorney may direct the physician not to release the x-rays, or the attorney may have taken the x-rays out of the doctor's office and retained them in his possession.

When the examiner is unable to easily obtain the x-ray films, he should note the importance of reviewing pertinent x-rays in his report, and request they be forwarded to him for review. The actual securing of x-rays is not his responsibility; by requesting them through the attorney who employed his services he is relieved of this obligation. He may defer his supplemental report until the x-rays are sent to him. A busy doctor in private practice does not have time to seek out x-rays in cases where opposing attorneys are uncooperative, and he should avoid these conflicts.

If the x-rays are available in a hospital or x-ray laboratory which the doctor visits frequently, it is a simple matter to obtain and review them. If necessary the physician should secure a written consent (utilizing a routine printed form) from the patient authorizing him to review the x-rays. Although this would usually have been obtained without difficulty on the patient's initial visit, it may be necessary to obtain the consent through the patient's attorney later. If the patient refuses permission to obtain the x-rays, this should be noted in the report and the matter can be resolved by the opposing lawyers.

The necessity of obtaining x-ray reports or actual x-ray films is an essential preliminary to treatment of injured persons; these patients may have received initial treatment in another facility such as a hospital emergency room or dispensary, then reported to a private doctor for follow-up care. Unfortunately some hospitals refuse to disclose any information without legal consent forms, especially if there is an accident with probable legal implications. The private doctor may be forced to repeat x-rays not only in order to treat the patient but also to protect himself from a possible malpractice suit. In this way he will be better equipped to justify his treatment of the patient later on when cross-examined at trial.

TESTIMONY—CONFLICT WITH MEDICAL CONVENTIONS AND VACATIONS

When the insurance company or attorney forwards a file of medical records to a physician preparatory to a defendant examination, the accompanying letter often indicates the date of the trial and requests the physician to acknowledge whether he will be able to testify if needed. Court calendars are usually set up to a year in advance, and sometimes the trial date may be several months distant. The physician may not have made plans to attend a medical convention or to take a vacation at that time, but he would be reluctant to exclude the possibility by committing himself to be present so far in advance. On the other hand, some cases are referred to the physician within a week or two of the trial date, after settlement conferences have failed, and here there is no problem as his travel schedule will probably already have been fixed. If the doctor does not believe he can be present for trial, he should not accept the referral, and should advise the defendant to arrange for another physician to examine the patient.

If the doctor has planned to attend a convention or take an extended vacation at the time the trial is to be held, he should notify the defendant of the probability of his absence at that time.

If the doctor's reputation as an expert witness is well established, the defendant may wish to reset the trial so that this particular physician can be called on to testify; or his examination and report may be all that will be required, as settlement of the case may be anticipated after receiving the expert's valued opinion. If the settlement for the defendant does not occur, however, his representatives can take the physician's deposition, but this is never as impressive as a personal appearance in court. Thus the decision whether to employ a medical examiner who may not be available for trial must be made by the defendant attorney, who is well aware of all facets of the case. If it is on the verge of settlement, he may still desire the examination, believing the negotiations will be quickly concluded once they have received a clear-cut, concise opinion from a recognized medical expert.

Absences for purposes of professional study or for a much needed vacation are to be expected. A competent medical specialist must keep abreast of recent developments by attending seminars and conventions. He cannot always plan a fixed schedule several months in advance, as some courses are announced only eight to ten weeks before. Should he arrange to attend a seminar, and subsequently be alerted for trial during the period he will be away, he is not positively bound to remain in town for the possibility of trial unless a valid subpoena is served upon him. As we indicated earlier, most of these cases are settled before trial, and some of the remainder are reset to a later date, or postponed a few days, so that only a small percentage actually do culminate in trial proceedings on the scheduled date. Understandably the doctor should not forego a chance for further medical education unless there are special circumstances about the case that justify a decision to remain available and on call.

It is very frustrating to a busy physician to postpone a vacation or convention trip for a trial alert, then have his services canceled at the last moment. Should be decide to go ahead with his trip, the defendant will undoubtedly be unhappy to learn that his doctor plans to be away at the time of trial; instead of taking his deposition, he may serve him with a subpoena to insure his court appearance.

Such an incident did occur in the case of an expert orthopaedist who was invited to participate as a panelist in a medical
seminar out of town on a day when he had previously been
alerted for trial (by an insurance company for whom he performed a large number of defense examinations). The defendant
attorney insisted upon the doctor's availability and delivered a
subpoena for his court appearance, following which the doctor
had no choice but to cancel his participation in the seminar. As
so often happens, the case was settled on the Friday afternoon
before the trial set on the following Monday; because the cancellation had occurred more than twenty-four hours before the
trial (although the interval was actually a week-end in which the
doctor's office was closed), no payment was made to the physician
to compensate him despite his full cooperation. It was too late for
him to participate in the medical seminar as a substitute panelist
had been secured, and furthermore his office schedule for the
following week had been filled after he had canceled plans to
be away.

Although the physician appreciated the uncertainties and unpredictable actions associated with negligence trials, he still believed that he had not received proper consideration for his
cooperation and for a while refused to accept further cases from
that insurance company. However, he later resumed cordial relationships after discussions with the claims manager. His services
were highly valued by all members of the firm and it was decided
to overlook the difficulty with the previous attorney who, as a
very aggressive and successful trial lawyer, wished to have all
available testimony to defend litigation. Both the attorney and
the physician had mutual respect for each other's ability, and they
resumed a good working relationship.

A recent ruling in the New York Superior Court that a physician may be excused from testifying or may ask for trial postponement in order to attend a medical convention, has already
been referred to in these pages. By this ruling (*Strakoski* vs
Bullock, 316, N.Y.S. 2d, 834—N.Y. Superior Court, App. Div.,
Nov. 5, 1970), the courts have recognized the need for continuing
education for physicians. Specifically, the New York Superior

Court ruled that the physician's attendance at a medical meeting justified delay of a trial and granting of a new trial date. This does not mean that all courts are bound by this ruling, but a physician could cite this in support of his request to be excused from attendance at a trial in conflict with his plans for post-graduate study or attendance at a medical convention. If the doctor has registered for the convention and has made hotel and travel reservations to attend it, he should use these facts to re-inforce his request to be excused from a court appearance. More-over, if he is a participant in the convention as a speaker or an exhibitor, his position will be further strengthened as he makes his request.

RELATIVE WEIGHT OF TESTIMONY OF SPECIALISTS

The testimony of a specialist carries more weight than medical evidence for the opposing side which is given by a physician less expert in the field of medicine under consideration. For example, if the plaintiff has a general practitioner or internist testifying about an orthopaedic condition, the jury may lend more credence to defendant testimony from a qualified orthopaedic expert. The attending doctor may be an excellent general physician, but he cannot qualify as an expert in a particular field in comparison to a Board-certified specialist.

In some instances the plaintiff's physician may be a friend of the specialist who is testifying for the defendant. In such cases, when asked to comment on the other doctor's qualifications, the doctor should answer that he is familiar with the doctor and con-siders him a competent physician in his particular field; or he may decline to answer, stating that he does not wish to make any comments, favorable or unfavorable, regarding another doc-tor's qualifications. Many presiding judges have ruled that it is not considered good professional ethics for one doctor to comment on the qualifications of another, and will permit the doctor to refrain from answering such questions.

In some instances the general practitioner or internist may be a physician who refers cases to the orthopaedic specialist, in which event the specialist obviously must use tact in his replies.

He may diplomatically point out that he knows the doctor well, as the doctor frequently refers cases to him for orthopaedic diagnosis and treatment. This will infer that the orthopaedist is better qualified to evaluate such injuries, and indicate to the jury that the plaintiff's doctor holds that particular expert in high esteem. This would certainly lend weight to the defendant testimony.

In one such instance the internist treated a husband and wife for osteoarthritis of the cervical spine and lumbar spine, with some improvement. However, the plaintiffs obviously were exaggerating their complaints, and would not recognize that the treatment had resolved the superimposed strain, leaving only the pre-existing arthritis. At the trial the defendant's orthopaedist testified that the osteoarthritis noted by x-ray was unchanged in its x-ray appearance before and after the accident; he stated there probably had been mild temporary aggravation of a pre-existing arthritic condition by a superimposed strain from the accident, but this was completely resolved when he examined the patients a year later. The treating doctor had recited the continuing complaints of both patients and diagnosed permanent disability for which periodic medical care would be needed indefinitely, as a direct result of the automobile accident. Because of the demonstrated gross exaggeration of symptoms and other evidence which questioned the veracity of the plaintiffs, a minimal verdict was returned for medical expenses and property damage only, despite clear liability.

The question as to which specialist's testimony should have more weight has been decided in several appellate court rulings. In a Workmen's Compensation case in Kentucky the question arose when there was conflicting testimony regarding the correct diagnosis in a case of chronic low back pain allegedly caused by an industrial injury. An orthopaedic surgeon diagnosed the condition as osteoarthritis rather than a herniated disc, whereas a radiologist who only interpreted the x-rays, did not believe there was sufficient evidence of arthritis on the films to account for the disability; he thought the symptoms could probably be attributed to nerve injury and pressure (rather unusual for one who never saw the patient). In this case the court correctly ruled that a clinical specialist would be more qualified to relate the disability to specific physiological changes than a radiologist.

In another Workmen's Compensation case in Louisiana the appellate court ruled that the opinion of a treating physician in close contact with a patient over a long period of time should have greater weight than the opinion of an equally qualified expert who did not have the benefit of repeated contact and examination. (See discussion under cross-examination. Page 307-311.) The court also noted that the testimony of a specialist with regard to matters falling within his specific field is entitled to greater weight than the general practitioner's testimony in the same matters.

TESTIMONY—FULL DISCLOSURE OF ALL EVIDENCE

The problem of full disclosure is a very controversial one which has its advocates and adversaries, and has often been discussed in medico-legal symposia. The problem is whether the physician (or any other witness) should voluntarily disclose every finding he has made, regardless of whether it is favorable or harmful to the side which has called him to the witness stand, or whether such information should be given only in response to specific questions. Another aspect of the same question is whether apparently irrelevant facts should be included in the doctor's report. Many attorneys contend that *all* facts should be reported, and the question of relevancy be left for the jury and court to decide.

In an actual occurrence reported in the AMA News 6/10/68 a pathologist failed to mention in his post mortem report that the deceased had an old appendectomy scar, completely unrelated to the litigation. Although the omission was definitely irrelevant, the plaintiff attorney confused the jury by his cross-examination of the pathologist, and even created considerable doubt as to whether the body discussed by the pathologist was really the same as the one under litigation. As a result the case was dismissed without going to the jury. For an attorney this may be considered clever legal tactics, but to most physicians these would not be in the least admirable, as justice was circumvented in this particular case on a technical point resulting from an irrelevant omission.

As a contrast, physicians have often been roughly cross-examined because of their inclusion of apparently irrelevant material in a physical examination. Here is another attempt to confuse the jury so as to depreciate the value of the doctor's testimony. For example, an orthopaedist, in reporting his examination for injuries to the neck and back, also included the blood pressure reading and the results of an examination of the ears, nose, mouth, throat, heart and lungs of the patient. This specialist had been trained to make a complete examination which, by the way, required only a few minutes more of his time and which sometimes resulted in disclosures of previously unidentified pathology. Thus the patient was always informed of any significant positive findings so that he could have proper treatment. And it was this careful, inclusive type of examination which the plaintiff attorney so sharply criticized in his cross-examination of the physician. Why? Because the doctor had involved himself in areas of the body that were not injured.

In his reply, the physician pointed out that hypertension is frequently associated with nervous individuals and could be responsible for many of the patient's subjective complaints, especially his anxiety manifestations and nervousness. He observed that in this particular case he had discovered significant hypertension which had been unrecognized and untreated by the patient's own physician. He also indicated that a chest examination may reveal medical conditions such as angina, coronary insufficiency, Pancoast tumor of the upper lobe of the lung, etc. any one of which can cause referred pain to the lower neck and left shoulder; none of these conditions are a result of accidental injury. In this case the effects of injury had completely cleared with no objective residuals. Before concluding that the patient was exaggerating his complaints, he wished to exclude non-traumatic diseases as a basis for them.

It would appear from the preceding incidents that the doctor can be in a quandary regarding the extent and completeness of his testimony. Clever attorneys try to confuse the medical witness and turn any omission or inclusion to their advantage; fair presentation of the facts for a just evaluation of the case appears to be of secondary interest to these lawyers. Occurrences of this nature often disillusion physicians as to the need and importance of medical testimony and make them unwilling to participate in additional cases.

An article by the eminent Melvin Belli in *Medical World News* maintained that the physician must divulge all the facts suggested by or relevant to the examiner's questions, otherwise he would be unfair to the court and jury and would cause a blemish upon the field of medicine in general. Common law justice depends upon the capacity of both advocates to bring out all the facts, although under the adversary proceeding each side attempts to demonstrate only the facts which are favorable to it. Belli raised the question whether a forensic physician can ethically hold back any facts or opinions not directly inquired of him.

He believes that the physician should volunteer any additional facts which may explain the situation, even though the question was not directly asked (probably because the attorney was not fully informed). He believes that the physician should be an advocate for justice, even if not solicited.

This view appears to be idealistic, as attorneys do not follow such a code and they do, time and again, withhold unfavorable facts, if at all possible. Belli points out that a mistrial or reversal may result if the medical expert consciously withholds evidence favorable to the other side. He believes that the medical expert who will admit nothing on cross-examination which detracts from his opinion, completely depreciates his testimony before lawyers, judge and jury. He further states that a more persuasive type of witness is one who is candid on cross-examination and does admit other possibilities, although he may testify that his opinion is the most reasonable conclusion.[2]

Belli's recommendations are not generally practiced. Most medical experts believe they should tell the truth and answer questions exactly as asked. They feel it is not their responsibility to volunteer information that was not asked of them. Actually when the doctor does volunteer information which is favorable to one side or the other, an objection is immediately raised by the other attorney and often sustained by the judge, who will then direct the witness to answer only what was asked and nothing more. This occurs daily in the courtroom and is definitely contrary to Belli's recommendation that the doctor should volunteer information. Most attorneys would react unfavorably if the volunteered information was detrimental to his cause. Of course the expert should not hide any information, and if asked a general question (such as availability of other tests which were not done in a particular case), he should answer to the best of his ability. Specifically he should reply to the questions put to him, and if the cross-examiner is not fully informed and does not ask the proper questions, it is *not* the responsibility of the medical expert to compensate for the ineptitude of the opposing counsel.

TESTIMONY ON BEHALF OF OPPOSING COUNSEL

There are times when the physician's testimony will be requested by the opposite side, i.e. other than the one for which he had performed the original examination. This commonly occurs when his report contains a fair and impartial evaluation of the case, which, however, is unfavorable to, or does not strengthen the evidence for, the side which requested his services. After the opposing attorney has received a copy of the physician's report, he may contact the doctor to learn whether he has been asked to testify in the case, realizing that because of his unfavorable report he may not be called as a witness by the litigant who originally requested his services. In this circumstance, the opposing lawyer will issue a subpoena to the doctor requiring him to be present in court, usually preceding this with a phone call or letter assuring him that he will be placed on telephone call and paid his usual fee as an expert witness. Not only is a subpoena necessary to insure his appearance, but it also relieves the doctor of any embarrassment in voluntarily appearing as an adverse witness against his patient or the defendant. Actually the doctor should *insist* upon a subpoena being served him if such a court appearance is requested. At trial he should testify in accordance with his report, but he should not amplify his statements except in response to the questions asked. He cannot be faulted if his testimony is adverse to the patient whom he examined and treated, or to the defendant who retained his services; however, he should confine himself to the questions asked, and not volunteer any additional information which might be damaging to the patient or defendant for whom he made the initial examination.

A recent example of this situation involved two attractive young girls who were referred by their attorney to an orthopaedist for evaluation of moderate injuries sustained two years previously. Both girls still had vague subjective complaints although they were working regularly and had not been under medical care for at least one year. The objective examination was completely negative and, in his report to their lawyer, the orthopaedist concluded that their complaints were probably due to a functional overlay with no residual organic disability.

As it happened, the doctor's testimony was requested by both the plaintiffs for whom he had made the evaluation, and also by the defendant attorney for whom he had made many defendant evaluations in the past. Thus he received a subpoena for his appearance from the defendant attorney, but he also received a subpoena from the plaintiff attorney. Under the circumstances he felt obligated to appear in court on behalf of the plaintiff; his testimony was given in an impartial manner. Despite the attractiveness of the girls the preponderantly male jury returned a defendant's verdict, and the doctor was unable to collect his fee for testimony from the plaintiffs; had he accepted the defendant's subpoena, his compensation would have been assured. However, he fully realized this contingency and believed his primary obligation was to his patients.

A physician with a large practice which includes both plaintiff and defendant patients, will occasionally be faced with situations of this type as a result of his impartial reports and basic objectivity. He should have no significant problem if he testifies in a detached manner for whoever requests his evidence and assumes the role of a medical witness seriously. This will enable him to carry out his obligation in a satisfactory and helpful manner.

INTERVENTION OF JUDGES

Although the judge's function in the trial is to preside over the court, to determine the law, and to see that the judicial forms are adhered to, there are occasions when the judge will intervene in the questioning of plaintiff or defendant medical witnesses. In the American judicial system, the function of the presiding judge is to pass upon questions of law and not upon the facts. The evaluation of the facts and establishment of their weight and veracity is within the province of the jury.

Most judges are neutral and adhere strictly to this policy. However, there is an occasional exception—a judge who will frequently interrupt the witness by either questioning a statement that has been made or interposing a question of his own in an attempt to clarify an obscure situation. At times this is helpful, but the witness may be unduly influenced by the judge's attitude and statements; the tenor and composition of the question and tone of voice frequently indicates to the witness the judge's frame of mind and opinion in the matter. A timid witness may be unwilling to continue to testify with the same trend of thought or to make a statement contradictory to the judge's apparent opinion. Although judicial intervention may provide grounds for appeal, it is not usually requested, as the appeal process is costly and delays are frequently lengthy. Thus, although the judge's intervention often is accepted without objection, there are occasionally reports of admonition by an appellate court to justices who make this a common practice.

A somewhat innocuous intervention was frequently noted in a suburban court during the qualification of an expert medical witness who was well known to the jurist. As the doctor began to recite his qualifications, the judge would stop him and state to the jury that this witness was well known to him as a specialist in orthopaedic surgery, well qualified in his field, and certainly able to render an opinion as a medical expert, followed by: "No further questions necessary regarding his qualifications, continue your inquiry." The counsel cannot then take time to demonstrate the impressive background and professional standing of his witness to the jury, as he dare not ask further questions regarding qualifications after such a statement from the bench.

Another example was seen in the District of Columbia courts where some judges would stop the witness in his testimony and rephrase his statements in words of their own choosing, then ask the witness if this was not what he meant. In one instance the doctor was differentiating the traumatic factor of persistent low back symptoms in a sixty-five year-old obese woman involved in a bus accident two years before, from osteoarthritis of the spine. He attributed half of her present symptoms to that accident as a result of traumatic aggravation, and the other half to her pre-existing arthritis and obesity. It was obviously impossible to give any type of mathematical formula with certainty, and in an effort to be fair the witness chose a path down the middle. However, the judge angrily interrupted the doctor with words to this effect, "I will not let you testify in that manner; are you trying to set the award for this court by telling us that half is due to the accident and another half is due to something else? You are obviously trying to set the monetary award in this case and I will not permit that. Doctor, aren't you really trying to say that the symptoms were precipitated by the accident, so that the onset of her back symptoms came at an earlier date and with more intensity than would have been anticipated without that accident?" This interpretation was also correct and the witness agreed with the judge, but later he did have a chance to indicate that he was not interested in the monetary award and was making no attempt in his testimony to influence that award.

In the same case, the plaintiff's counsel attempted to show that his expert witness was also a regular examiner for the Transit Company and was frequently used as their own expert witness, in order to augment the impact of his evidence. This type of questioning is usually used by attorneys against experts for the defense to demonstrate probable prejudice against plaintiffs and to depreciate the value of their testimony. The judge objected to the question and would not permit an answer. In situations like the preceding, the doctor must *keep his cool* and remember that he cannot prevail over the judge. Should he answer the judge's inquiry unfavorably and strongly disagree with him, he may have further problems with that jurist before he steps down from the witness box. Wherever possible he should agree or point out in a respectful manner any variations of his opinion, and perhaps later bring out additional points, through questions from his own counsel. Any direct conflict of the witness with the presiding judge may react unfavorably upon the jury.

IMPARTIAL MEDICAL TESTIMONY

Some jurisdictions have set up panels for impartial medical testimony by medical experts, in an effort to overcome the problems arising when medical evidence is presented through partisan experts hired by parties to lawsuits. Although these panels have been tried in several jurisdictions, they have not achieved general acceptance in the adversary system of justice now prevailing in this country. It is difficult to have both litigants agree upon a neutral medical expert and abide by his opinion. Although there have been various modifications of the practice of setting up such a panel in several jurisdictions in the United States, it has met with only limited success.

The usual procedure is about as follows: after an impartial medical expert has expressed his opinion prior to the trial proceedings, the concerned parties are often brought to a settlement conference. If the case proceeds to litigation, the medical expert may or may not be asked to testify, depending on the agreement made at the time of his employment. Usually a subpoena is not required. In addition, it is generally recommended that the expert have no pre-trial conference with the attorney requesting his presence in court.

A project was set up in New York City in 1952 with one hundred and fifty specialists, and the same arrangement has also been tried in Illinois and California. To describe the New York project further: in 1967 Edward Aarons[1] reported that a panel of impartial medical experts had been operating successfully in New York City, and that in fifteen years 1247 cases had been settled out of court, representing 80 per cent of those with disputed medical evidence. State Supreme Court Justice Emilio Nunez favorably endorsed this system, stating that it frequently avoids the courtroom spectacle of two doctors presenting diametrically opposed testimony, which always causes a poor image for the medical profession.

The opponents of the above system believe that the doctor (described as an "impartial medical expert") is given an unwarranted halo of authority; although he is still subject to personal impressions, he is elevated to an authority status to decide disputed medical evidence. However, on the "plus" side in this debate, there is little question that the number of court appearances required of doctors treating personal injury cases is definitely limited by the use of an impartial medical witness panel, thereby avoiding considerable loss of these doctors' time for on-call status and testimony. The system also protects patients from the strain of prolonged litigation, which often runs for years and results in aggravation of emotional stress produced by the prolonged delay. This is particularly true of the apprehensive individual with exaggerated complaints.

The selection of the panel is of utmost importance and must be done with great discretion. In New York a joint committee was established within the New York City Academy of Medicine and the State Medical Society to select the panel. The members of this committee eliminate from consideration doctors who make frequent court appearances or have extensive association with insurance companies or industrial clinics. The doctors selected are called in rotation, usually no more than three or four times a year. They are paid a standard fee for the consultation from a fund administered by the court and derived through the budget of the city government.

The presence of the impartial medical witness panel also has a definite prophylactic value, as the average physician does not wish to submit an unsubstantiated medical report which may be completely rejected as false and misleading. He will exercise caution and restraint in his reports, realizing that his opinions may be contradicted by an impartial expert and result in considerable personal embarrassment. This factor alone results in a higher rate of settlement and diminished use of the impartial expert.

Despite the successful use of the panel in New York City, few other areas have adopted the system, largely because of the objections of plaintiff attorneys who find that the impartial expert panel reduces the amount of recovery in many of their cases. A plaintiff's attorney usually is able to find some physician who will cooperate with him and write the type of report he desires, in an effort to obtain as much money as possible out of the case. The impartial medical panel would soon render such reports worthless, and this is fully realized by lawyers specializing in negligence cases. Some defendant attorneys also object to the impartial panel on the grounds that they may be forced into settling some cases which they believe they could successfully defend if the unimpeachable aura of the impartial expert had not been injected into the case.

SUBPOENA FOR
DEPOSITION

A deposition may be taken of either the plaintiff's or de-fendant's doctor by either litigant, for purposes of discovery of information or in lieu of court testimony, if the witness will be out of town on the trial date, but evidence by deposition is never as effective as live testimony. Either attorney may wish to learn the nature of the physician's testimony in advance of the trial, in order to better prepare his case and determine his objectives and trial technique. It will also aid the attorney when he confers with his own medical expert before trial; the doctor can interpret the medical data and prepare the attorney for cross-examination of the opposing witness.

Depositions are generally taken in the doctor's office at his convenience, but not necessarily so. The opposing attorney may subpoena the witness to give his deposition in the attorney's office at a designated time, but if he wishes a cooperative witness, the lawyer usually accedes to the doctor's preference as to loca-tion and time. There is no set fee for a deposition other than the subpoena fee for an ordinary witness, which will prevail unless the physician is knowledgeable enough to demand compensation as an expert. This should be agreed upon in advance by a frank discussion between the attorney and witness. In some instances the physician should insist upon payment in advance, before the deposition begins, as an occasional unscrupulous lawyer may tender only the ordinary witness fee after conclusion of the proceeding, especially if the evidence given by the witness is unfavorable to his client. Although more informal, a deposition is conducted under court rules of evidence; objections noted are subject to ruling by the judge when the deposition is read in court in lieu of testimony. Off-record remarks are permitted.

Upon receiving a subpoena for a deposition from the opposing attorney, the doctor should immediately contact the attorney who employed his services and request guidance. In many instances the deposition can be arranged by mutual agreement of defendant and plaintiff attorneys, without need of a subpoena, at the convenience of the medical witness. However, the attorney to whom the doctor submitted his report may desire a conference with his doctor before the deposition in order to instruct him and prepare him for anticipated questions.

Many cases are settled after deposing the opposing medical witnesses; the plaintiff or defendant attorney may then learn for the first time of unanticipated opinions or facts which are grossly detrimental to their case and may lead to an unfavorable jury verdict.[12]

The following incident represents an attempt to subpoena a defendant's physician to take his deposition prior to trial in a town sixty miles away in another state. The orthopaedist had previously examined the plaintiff in a Virginia hospital by special appointment. Ten days before trial the plaintiff attorney decided to take the deposition of the defendant's witness and issued a subpoena for his appearance at his office some sixty miles distant. The defendant attorney learned of this maneuver and promptly warned the doctor of the forthcoming subpoena. The subpoena could not be served, as the doctor did not have an office in that state and made only occasional visits to the hospital in that area. The sheriff's office contacted the physician by phone to learn when he would appear in the state so that the subpoena could be properly served; he was politely informed of the circumstances of the subpoena, and it was suggested that he return it to the plaintiff attorney as the doctor had no plans to return to that state until the date of trial. The sheriff's deputy also informed the doctor that there was no check attached to the subpoena for his witness fee or to reimburse him for his travel. The doctor erroneously believed that this would have invalidated the subpoena even if it had been served, but he later learned that although this was the law in the District of Columbia, it was not the case in Virginia. However, the unpleasant situation was easily avoided as the doctor was careful not to cross the state line at that time.

An incident in which a subpoena for a deposition was served upon a medical expert who had made a defendant examination is illustrated in the following case. The right of a medical expert to protect the value of his expert opinions was supported by the judicial action that arose out of this deposition. It has long been held that the opposing counsel does not have the right to *pick the brains* of a medical expert by issuing a subpoena, without adequate and reasonable compensation. In this case, the plaintiff had been treated by a competent orthopaedic surgeon who had made a fair evaluation and had written a reasonable medical report in which he noted that the patient had made a satisfactory recovery. Later, another orthopaedist who had treated the patient gave a less favorable prognosis. The report of the defendant's expert supported the findings of the initial treating orthopaedist.

Two weeks before trial the defendant's medical expert received a subpoena without an accompanying fee, at his Maryland office, served in the proper manner and personally delivered, requiring him to appear for a deposition the following week at the plaintiff attorney's office in Rockville, Maryland (approximately twenty miles from the doctor's office). The doctor could not attend at the time requested as he had surgery scheduled at exactly that hour; he phoned the attorney and arrangements were made to take his deposition later that afternoon, following surgery.

The deposition was also attended by the attorney represent-

ing the defendant. The doctor was sworn in but no effort was
made to qualify him as a medical expert. He was asked to hand
over his medical records to the plaintiff's attorney who perused
these records in detail. The attorney selected a copy of the
medical report, which had already been forwarded to both
the defendant and plaintiff attorneys, and the front sheet of his
medical records on which the patient's name, address and a brief
history were recorded. These were identified as exhibits in a
formal manner, with some apparent effort to impress the witness
with the gravity of these routine records.

The doctor had made some hand-written penciled notes in
the margin of his copy of the medical report, after reviewing
his own records and the reports of the plaintiff's physicians, in
preparation for the forthcoming trial. The plaintiff's attorney
requested the doctor to read these notes into the record; the
witness declined, stating that these notes represented an interpretation of the medical records of the plaintiff and of his own
records, resulting in an opinion regarding the patient's medical
condition. He further stated that he had appeared in response
to a subpoena as an ordinary witness, and no arrangements had
been made for his testimony as a medical expert. The plaintiff
attorney repeated his request, but the doctor again declined.
At this point, the plaintiff attorney abruptly terminated the
deposition and stated that he would file a motion in court to
compel the witness to answer the questions. He also stated that
he would request attorney fees for filing the motion to compel the
witness to answer—these fees to be paid by the medical witness.

The whole situation appeared to be ironical, inasmuch as the
medical witness had not been paid to attend the deposition, not
even for his transportation for the forty-mile roundtrip from his
office, in addition to cancellation of some two and a half hours of
office appointment time. He was astounded to learn that there
was a possibility that he would be required to pay a fee of fifty
dollars to the opposing attorney, in addition to disruption of his
professional schedule to attend a deposition required by the legal
proceedings.

The plaintiff attorney filed the following motion to compel an answer by the defendant's physician. This was heard in Circuit Court in Montgomery County, Maryland before Judge Joseph Mathias.

MOTION TO COMPEL ANSWER UPON ORAL EXAMINATION

Barbara Q. Campbell, by her attorneys, Schwartz and Mooney, respectfully moves the Court to enter an order directing Milton J. Crisp, M.D. to answer questions he refused to answer upon his oral examination in this case upon the following grounds:

1. This action by plaintiff is a personal injury claim for injuries sustained in an automobile accident.

2. This court directed plaintiff to submit to an examination by Dr. Crisp, the physician selected by the defendant.

3. On June 15, 1972, in the office of Schwartz and Mooney at 4 o'clock p.m., a time and place agreed upon by stipulation of witness and counsel for both parties, the oral examination of Dr. Crisp was commenced.

4. A subpoena had been served upon Dr. Crisp requiring him to bring to the deposition all of his reports and office notes concerning his examination of plaintiff.

5. At his oral examination, Dr. Crisp produced plaintiff's exhibit No. 2, upon which he had made some hand-written notes concerning plaintiff.

6. Both counsel for plaintiff and counsel for defendant were unable to read the notes of Dr. Crisp written as aforesaid, and Dr. Crisp was asked to interpret his writing on plaintiff's exhibit No. 2.

7. Dr. Crisp refused to answer as to what his handwritten notes said, claiming he was entitled to an expert witness fee.

8. The information sought by plaintiff on the oral examination of Dr. Crisp related to whatever he had previously written and under no circumstances could this be considered a request by plaintiff for the doctor to express an opinion. Even if the handwritten notes contained an opinion, plaintiff is entitled to examine Dr. Crisp about any opinions he had already expressed.

9. For the foregoing reasons, plaintiff requests that this Court order be issued and directs Milton J. Crisp, M.D. to attend the resumption of his deposition and answer questions which he refused to answer on his oral examination commenced June 15, 1972, and that attorney's fees in the sum of Fifty Dollars for having necessitated this motion be lodged against Dr. Crisp.

Schwartz and Mooney
Attorneys for Plaintiff

The defendant's attorney filed the following opposition to the plaintiff's motion.

OPPOSITION TO PLAINTIFF'S MOTION TO COMPEL ANSWER UPON ORAL EXAMINATION

Comes now the defendant, Thomas C. McPherson, by and through his attorneys, Miltner and Morton, and respectfully moves his Honorable Court to deny the plaintiff's motion to compel answers upon oral examination and for reasons states:

1. This is an action by the plaintiff for a personal injury claim for injuries sustained in an automobile accident.

2. This court directed the plaintiff to submit to an examination by Dr. Milton J. Crisp, the examining physician selected by the defendant.

3. On June 15, 1972, in the law office of Schwartz and Mooney, at 4 o'clock p.m., the time and place agreed upon by stipulation of witness and counsel for both parties, the oral examination of Dr. Crisp was commenced.

4. Upon his oral examination, Dr. Crisp was asked to interpret notations which he had made in the margin of the plaintiff's exhibit No. 2, concerning the plaintiff's medical condition.

5. Dr. Crisp refused to interpret said notations indicating that such interpretation would be in the nature of expert testimony, for which he was not being compensated.

6. Such notations recorded by a doctor in the course of medical examination are the product of the exercise of that individual's faculties as an expert. As such, they are in the nature of property and within the protection of constitutional guarantees against taking thereof without just compensation.

7. Dr. Crisp, having used his scientific and technical knowledge in the defense's examination of the plaintiff, is now being asked by the plaintiff to render an expert medical opinion without the normal expert witness compensation.

8. An expert witness is not required, without just compensation, to translate, interpret, or evaluate any notes which he has made pursuant to a medical examination and which constitute memoranda of his medical opinion formulated at the time of the examination. The disclosure of the content of handwritten notations of a physician would require an expression of the expert opinion represented by such notations, for which the expert must be compensated.

9. For the foregoing reasons, it is requested that the defendant's motion to compel answers of Dr. Crisp upon oral examination without compensation be denied. Additionally, it is requested that

reasonable attorney's fees for the preparation of this opposition be lodged against the plaintiff.

Miltner and Morton
Attorneys for Defendant

At the hearing, the court ruled in favor of the medical witness and denied the motion to compel an answer upon oral examination, supporting the witness' contention that he had not been compensated as a medical expert. The plaintiff's attorney then asked for permission to continue the deposition that same afternoon (a Friday); this would have been a severe imposition upon the medical expert, as he had a heavily loaded office schedule which could not have been canceled at such a late hour. The attorney wished to complete the deposition as the trial was scheduled for the following Monday; this request was denied. Thereupon, the plaintiff attorney requested dismissal of the case on a non-suit basis; this was granted. The court also directed the plaintiff to pay the defendant's attorney fees in the amount of one hundred dollars for opposing the motion to compel the medical witness to answer the questions arising in this deposition.*

This case substantiates the position that a medical expert cannot be deposed as a medical expert without adequate compensation. The question frequently arises but it is seldom decided in the courtroom. This case adds another decision which supports the value of expert medical testimony.† The payment of attorney's fees for opposing the plaintiff motion should also act as a deterrent in future similar situations in which the witness had a just and substantial basis for his refusal to answer the oral examination, and in which the witness was not capricious, arbitrary, or unreasonable in his position.

DEPOSITION USED FOR HARASSMENT

Depositions are ordinarily used for purposes of discovery of evidence or to substitute for testimony when the witness cannot

---

Crown vs McDonald, No. 34,083, Sixth Judicial Circuit for Maryland, 6-23-72.

†*Wilson vs Baltimore Transit Co., Superior Court of Baltimore City,* G. J. Nyles; Daily Record, May 7, 1958.

be present at trial. The following incident demonstrates an extraordinary motive for a deposition: to harass a medical expert. Any physician with a well established reputation as a witness, for either the defendant or the plaintiff, is subject to harassment and attempts to depreciate his testimony through apparent prejudices or identification as a professional medico-legal witness. It is paradoxical that the physician who does express an interest in medico-legal matters is often severely attacked in the legal proceedings. When his colleagues learn of such harsh treatment, it limits the number of physicians who wish to engage in medico-legal practice. One of the purposes of this publication is to disseminate practical knowledge of medico-legal procedures so that physicians can participate more intelligently and efficiently in negligence litigation in which their services are required. Paradoxically, the physician who does become an expert in this field feels the brunt of attacks in an attempt to dissuade him from further participation. Nevertheless, the alert physician will recognize these attacks for what they are—merely harassment to increase financial gain for the attorney.

In the following example a subpoena was received by an orthopaedic expert approximately one month before trial.

IN THE CIRCUIT COURT FOR MONTGOMERY COUNTY, MARYLAND

JAMES ALLEN, et al.	)	
Plaintiffs	)	
vs.	)	Law No. 61,841
EDWARD JENKINS, et al.	)	
Defendant	)	

NOTICE FOR DEPOSITION

The plaintiffs, pursuant to the Maryland Rules of Procedure, will take the deposition of John Davidson, M.D., 501 Indian Head Highway, Oxon Hill, Maryland, at 10:00 A.M., on Friday, August 20, 1971, at the offices of Andrew Hale, Esq., 788 Pershing Drive, Silver Spring, Maryland, before Jane Clark, Notary Public, Locust Road, Silver Spring, Maryland, or some officer duly authorized to administer an oath, *to continue from day to day until completed;* said

Dr. Davidson is to bring with him to the deposition *all appointment books and all billing records since January 1, 1970, and copies of all reports rendered in third-party liability cases since that time.* [Emphasis by author.]

SLOAN AND BROOK

By _____

William Sloan
608 Parkview Lane
Takoma Park, Md.
PO 1-2640
Attorneys for Plaintiffs

The subpoenaed physician had testified a year previously for the defendant in a trial involving the same litigants, resulting in a directed verdict for the defendant. However, the case was appealed on a technicality, and was to be re-tried approximately a month after the date set for his deposition. There was a complete transcript available of his testimony from the previous trial so that there was no need for a deposition for purposes of discovery; in fact the summons made specific reference to facts relating to the doctor's type of practice rather than to the case to be litigated. The doctor had two practices, one in suburban Maryland and one in downtown Washington; the subpoena required him to bring to the lawyer's suburban office all office records, bills, appointment books, billing records and copies of all reports rendered in medico-legal matters for the previous one and a half years. The doctor did not maintain a separate file for medico-legal cases; in order to comply with the subpoena it would have been necessary for the doctor or his assistants to review all records for the previous one and a half years, selecting several hundreds of plaintiff and defendant cases which had either been examined or treated by him. This would have required at least one week's work, and the material would have filled approximately ten file drawers. In addition the clinical records would have been privileged inasmuch as they pertained to other patients, and many were kept in another city (the downtown Washington office), outside the jurisdiction of the subpoena.

The doctor did not report for the deposition but instead notified his attorney, who promptly filed a motion at the courthouse to quash the subpoena on the grounds that it was unreasonable and not pertinent to the case under litigation. The motion was granted and the doctor heard nothing more of the incident until the case came to trial. It was settled on the day before trial for a relatively small sum. Incidentally, no fee was offered by the plaintiff attorney to compensate the physician for the deposition or for the even greater expense of transporting the many file cases to the deposition twenty miles away.

It was apparent that this maneuver was an extraordinary effort to harass an opposing witness on the part of a vengeful, unscrupulous attorney who had little or no respect for professional colleagues.

8 CROSS-EXAMINATION

Cross-examination refers to the questioning of a witness by the opposing counsel after he has given direct testimony. The purpose may be either to diminish the effect of his previous testimony or to develop pertinent evidence that was omitted in the direct examination. The opposing defense counsel may possess information that has not yet been placed in evidence, such as previous injuries and accidents, and he may state these in a hypothetical question in an effort to alter the stated opinion of the plaintiff's witness after being furnished all the facts in the case.

BASIS AND TECHNIQUES

The length and intensity of the the examination depends on what evidence the doctor has given in response to questioning by the attorney who called him to court. If he has testified fairly and given acceptable answers consistent with the facts and medical knowledge, the cross-examination is often brief or may even be waived. But if he has demonstrated that he is partisan or an advocate, by exaggerating the facts or offering improbable answers not logically related to the facts, or has over-treated the patient and rendered an unrealistic bill for his professional services, he will undoubtedly be subjected to a thorough grilling by the opponent's attorney. A smart trial attorney eagerly awaits such prey, as this gives him the opportunity to deflate his opponent's case by demonstrating the inconsistencies and partiality of one of their key witnesses. The medical witness plays a major role in a personal injury action; the manner in which he gives his evidence will have a significant effect on the outcome of the litigation.

279

The manner of cross-examination often varies with the quali-fications of the witness. A family physician with little expertise is usually treated gently unless he grossly exaggerates the facts or submits an unwarranted bill. A medical expert, such as an orthopaedist or neurosurgeon, may be questioned longer and more intensely on cross-examination than in his direct testimony, as his evidence is given more weight and may have more in-fluence on the final decision of the court.

Occasionally the opposing attorney may use a witness to corroborate evidence already given by his physician; if he is suc-cessful, this will increase the weight of such evidence, as it is an admission from the other side. If the expert has a reputation of fairness and objectivity, he may try to get into evidence several points he forgot to ask his witness who has already been excused.

On the other hand, if the witness has not damaged his case to any significant extent, or has a reputation for shrewdness under cross examination, he may be asked only a few non-vital ques-tions (to justify his bill!) or nothing at all. The smart attorney will realize that the cross-examination may open up new areas previously denied during direct testimony, or give the witness the opportunity to re-emphasize significant evidence which will then be strongly impressed upon the jury. The court-wise expert witness will seize upon any opening to elaborate on the question asked, and perhaps get into evidence several facts he forgot to mention during his direct examination. In addition he may reply in such a manner that his attorney will *get the message* or recog-nize an opportunity to emphasize certain facts when the cross-examiner has finished and he is allowed his *re-direct* examination. He should not arrange for signals to his attorney to call his atten-tion to the need for emphasis of points brought out by the cross-examiner, as this may be spotted and the witness exposed as an advocate. If his attorney is not clever enough to recognize the opportunities to enhance his case, that is his problem and his loss; the medical witness is there to help him, but not to be his co-counsel.

A good example involves presentation of the medical history. A defendant examiner who sees the patient only for the purpose of evaluation and not for treatment, often cannot testify regarding history if the opposing attorney objects. He can only state the results of his physical examination, x-rays, and opinion. However, if the opposing attorney asks questions which relate to the history, such as, "Did Mr. B tell you he had numbness in his left arm?" or, "Did Mr. B complain to you about persistent pain in his lower back?"—then he has opened up the subject, and the court will permit the witness to give the full medical history if the other attorney asks for it on his re-direct examination.

Cross-examination is an important means of separating truth from falsehood and reducing the effects of exaggerated statements, according to Attorney William J. Stewart of Washington, D. C. (now a Superior Court Justice) in a symposium on the role of cross-examination. He believes it is indispensable to the adversary system of justice. He stressed that the lawyer adopts the cause of his client and undertakes to present that cause in its most favorable light, by magnifying his own arguments and minimizing those of his opponent. He observed that medicine has some scientific basis for presentation of medical facts, whereas the lawyer must rely upon the oath of the witness to tell the truth; this is the reason cross-examination is so important.[33]

Should the doctor, during the cross-examination, be given new information of which he was not aware when he made his medical examination and diagnoses, he should evaluate it impartially when asked questions based on the additional history. This impartiality is particularly needed with regard to previous accidents, injuries or litigation, if the patient did not previously give the treating physician a complete history and background of his condition. Such information is often discovered by the defendant by consulting various references available to him, such as a Central Accident Index. If the doctor has testified on the basis that there was no previous injury or difficulty in the area injured in the accident now under litigation, and is thereafter confronted on cross-examination with evidence of previous similar difficulty, of other accidents, hospitalizations, treatment, etc., he should consider the effect of this new evidence on the opinion he expressed in court earlier; he should not be reluctant to change that opinion if indicated. In no instance should the doctor support a patient who has been dishonest and has withheld pertinent information. He should demonstrate his impartiality by his willingness to change his opinion based on the additional information supplied during his testimony. However, if the doctor honestly believes additional information does not change the validity of his previously expressed opinion, he should state this. The point here is that the medical witness should not make any attempt to cover up for a patient who has misled him and placed him in an embarrassing position. The doctor who is willing to change his opinion based on new facts gains stature and his entire testimony becomes more impressive to the jury and court, whereas the doctor who refuses to change his opinion despite gross evidence contrary to his stated opinion, loses credibility.

The doctor is testifying as an impartial witness and not as an advocate; nevertheless he will find that the opposing counsel should be regarded as just that—an opponent, no matter how friendly he may seem. There is no reason for fear or apprehension if the doctor remembers that he is being questioned in his own field; the doctor has infinitely more knowledge of medicine than the attorney can obtain by study and preparation for the trial. Nevertheless, the doctor will also find that many astute attorneys do study assiduously for their trial and *bone up* on one particular subject as the nature of the case warrants; their questions are often quite pertinent and reflect a clear understanding of the subject in controversy.

Under cross-examination the physician should anticipate the paths down which the opposing attorney is attempting to lead him, probably in a maneuver to secure an answer which was not given in direct testimony. The experienced physician can often anticipate the answers the cross-examiner desires, be guided accordingly, and thus avoid being trapped in an indefensible position.

If the physician is not thoroughly familiar with the topics likely to be discussed, it would be wise to review recent literature or authoritative text books prior to trial. In any event, he should be thoroughly cognizant of the anatomy of the area under discussion (for example, the composition and nerve distribution of the brachial plexus), as frequently the attorney will attempt to deflate his testimony by pointing out errors or lack of knowledge on some minor point in anatomy, in order to diminish the doctor's image before the jury. When in doubt, the physician should answer in general terms, avoiding specific points; this may suffice to get him *off the hook*.

If the doctor is completely unaware of an answer to a particular question, he should not *bluff* but honestly state that he does not recall it at the moment; he can then add that he has text books readily available for reference when needed, and that he often uses them instead of trying to retain everything in his memory. Such an answer is preferable to an erroneous answer which may lead him into a trap. Most professional men frequently consult texts and references for exact technical knowledge. Surely it is also not an admission of ignorance, when you are questioned in this way, to indicate that your opinion is not absolutely conclusive.

RECOGNITION OF TEXT BOOKS AS AUTHORITIES

The physician does not necessarily have to recognize any one text as an authority; he can disagree with the so-called authorities if he is convinced they are wrong and he has a sound basis for disagreement. Certainly there is no greater authority than he regarding that particular patient, whom he has examined and the text book has not! He should also be alert for partial quotations from books or articles which may give an improper or incomplete connotation. When in doubt, he should ask to see the source and review the preceding and following paragraphs or pages. If the entire passage is read, it may become apparent that the brief quotation made by the opposing counsel does not reflect the true opinion of the author, which may have been taken out of context. The witness should remember that once he admits the authority of a book or article, he may be subjected to examination on the contents of that text. As a matter of fact, courts have ruled that textbooks of established repute can be offered in evidence even though the witness refuses to recognize the authority or to acknowledge familiarity with its contents (*Abrams* vs. *Gordon,* U.S. District Court for D. C., 1959; Court of Appeals, 1960).

Each witness will probably develop his own response to the question of recognition of the expertise of a particular author. One elderly orthopaedist, with many decades of experience as a defendant examiner and witness, was particularly effective in parrying this type of cross-examination. When the cross-examining attorney would read a portion of a textbook which was contradictory to the doctor's opinion expressed on direct examination, the exchange would go somewhat in this fashion. The attorney would ask him whether he recognized the expertise of the author and the validity of the opinion expressed, to which the doctor would respond, "Son, I don't know the gentleman, but since he is a doctor and obviously has the time and ability to write a book, I am sure he is a fine gentleman, most likely *holed up* in a nice university, teaching medical students. On the other hand, the opinion I have expressed in this case is simply and solely based upon my experiences in the examination and treatment of patients in my office, and knowledge gained in the operating room. I invite you to choose which opinion has the most merit in this particular case." Suffice it to say the same lawyer never confronted this physician twice with the same question!

Under no circumstances should the physician lose his temper and appear sarcastic or angry, as this is often a trick to entice him to make statements which he may later regret.

When the opposing attorney has been unable to attack the direct testimony, he may ask whether the doctor is being paid to testify or to try to show that the fees are exhorbitant or unjustified; this is usually a sign that the witness has done very well in his testimony and the cross-examiner is resorting to desperate methods to reduce its value. There is no reason not to disclose that the doctor expects to be paid, as everyone else in the courtroom also is being paid for their time, including professional witnesses called by the other side. If no fee has been determined, the doctor may respond frankly that he expects to be paid for the amount of time involved in the court appearance and the loss of time from his practice; he should also state that his charges are not contingent upon the outcome of the litigation. If the fee has been agreed upon in advance, he may state it if no objections have been raised by his attorney.[12]

INCONSISTENCY OF TESTIMONY WITH PREVIOUS TESTIMONY OR MEDICAL PUBLICATIONS OF WITNESS

The medical specialist's role as an expert witness is not always a pleasant one. Although most lawyers are respectful and courteous to a professional witness, there are a few enterprising, zealous members of the bar who will stop at nothing in order to obtain a larger recovery for their client—and themselves. Sometimes an opposing attorney of this type will attack the medical witness in an attempt to prejudice the jury against him by defaming his character, demonstrating alleged inconsistencies in previous testimony, attempting to label him as a professional witness who is constantly in court, calling attention to inconsistencies in his testimony with that given in other trials, or between his testimony and his medical publications. Such tactics often have a reverse effect on the jury, if the medical witness replies calmly and concisely with accurate facts which refute the allegations. Occasionally the presiding judge may interfere and stop an unwarranted attack on the reputation of a member of another respected profession. If there is no rule on witnesses, a physician waiting to testify for the opposite side may be in the audience and hear the abusive tactics of his attorney. This may have an adverse effect on him, in sympathy for an unwarranted attack on a medical colleague; after witnessing the uncalled-for attack he may be less enthusiastic in his testimony and refuse to substantiate vital facts, resulting in a lower verdict.

A prominent physician who has published medical papers, books, or monographs, may be questioned on any of his medical writings. The opposing attorney often attempts to downgrade the witness and his authenticity, by demonstrating that testimony in this particular case is at variance with what he has written in medical articles. He should be cognizant of his personal medical literature, particularly when testifying in a case which involves a subject on which he has written. For example, if he has written about knee injuries and he is testifying in a case which involves such an injury, it may be helpful to review that article, as the opposing attorney may refer to this in his cross-examination. The doctor should recognize that the attorney is attempting to trap him. He should follow the same line of thought as in his article, and in this way avoid the embarrassment that would follow if he disagreed with himself.

An example of this maneuver is demonstrated in the case of a young female injured in an automobile accident with multiple injuries. Several months later an orthopaedist discovered a marked laxity of the anterior cruciate ligament of her left knee. Although the patient had no significant complaints about the left knee and had not received any specific treatment, the treating physician related these findings to the automobile accident. The orthopaedist must have known that a rupture of the anterior cruciate ligament of this magnitude would have resulted in a large hemarthrosis into the knee joint, which would have caused immediate disability and required aspiration of the joint and either splinting or cast immobilization. In this case the patient had no arthrocentesis and no immobilization whatsoever, not even an elastic bandage support. She denied any previous injury, but it was obvious that there must have been some previous difficulty. There was also some laxity of the opposite knee ligaments, although to a lesser extent. Congenital ligamentous laxity is well recognized but in this case there was considerable disparity between the two knees, which usually is not the case if the condition is congenital in origin.

The treating orthopaedist did not testify in accordance with these obvious facts, although they must have been just as apparent to him as to the defendant's examiner. He apparently realized that such testimony would severely damage the plaintiff's case, as she was trying to establish damages based on permanent disability. When the defendant orthopaedist did bring out these salient points, the plaintiff's attorney angrily attacked the physician's credibility and integrity.

The defendant's physician had observed that the function of her injured cruciate ligament was compensated for by an over-developed quadriceps mechanism; actually the left lower thigh was greater in circumference than the uninjured side. The doctor further testified that it was his belief that there had been a previous injury to this knee which the patient refused to admit.

In the cross-examination the patient's lawyer quoted from a monograph written by the testifying physician regarding knee injuries, which the lawyer alleged was inconsistent with his testimony. The article stated that it was rare to achieve full recovery after cruciate ligament rupture, even with a properly supervised program of rehabilitation and the full cooperation of the patient; it also stated that operative repair of the ruptured ligament is technically difficult and does not always assure an excellent result. In this particular case the patient cooperated with a progressive resistance exercise regime, and she did have a good result with minimal disability. Obviously all patients do not follow the textbook pattern; medical articles refer to the majority of cases but there are exceptions. The doctor indicated that he had *not* written that it was *impossible,* only *unusual* to obtain an excellent result after a severe cruciate ligament injury of the knee. He also stated that another reason for her recovery may have been that the initial injury had occurred long before this accident, and that over a prolonged period she had developed adequate compensation by her well-developed quadriceps muscu-lature.

Despite the medical testimony, the jury did award the plain-tiff one hundred thousand dollars, as there was clear liability as well as evidence of other minor injuries and scars beside the knee injury. This verdict was set aside by the court and the case was subsequently re-tried. The discussion regarding the medical writings and the reported findings on her knee were given much less attention at the second trial, the attorney apparently having recognized a formidable adversary from the previous cross-examination. This trial ended in an award to the plaintiff of twenty-five thousand dollars, a substantial amount for a case in which the major injury undoubtedly had occurred prior to the accident being litigated.

Subsequently the orthopaedist testified in another state. During the cross-examination by another attorney he was asked whether he kept two sets of records, one for testifying, and another in which he retained other memoranda and notes regarding his examinations which would be injurious to the defendant's cause and which he omitted from his file when he came to court. The witness testified that he did not keep two sets of records; he stated that he used a dictaphone when he made his examination and dictated his findings as the examination proceeded, except for his diagnosis and conclusions which were dictated after the patient left the room. All other information, including the history and examination, was dictated in front of the patient and there were no other notes made. The cross-examiner continued to question the doctor about "double records." At this point, the presiding judge, a stern jurist well known for his rugged individuality and strict disciplinary control of his courtroom, demanded that the cross-examiner produce the evidence which would substantiate his defamation of the character of a professional witness. The attorney was informed that he would not be permitted to continue unless he had definite and conclusive evidence which would demonstrate that the doctor was unethical or which would prejudice his character and credibility as a witness.

The plaintiff's attorney then produced a transcript of the previous trial regarding the knee injury and its discussion of the apparent discrepancy between the doctor's article and his testimony in that case. The attorney had not marked his place in the text and fumbled about for a few moments; he then questioned the witness whether he had testified in the knee injury case in Smithville a year before, and also if it were true that he had testified to a diagnosis and prognosis which did not agree with his previously published monograph. The judge then intervened and asked the attorney to state the relationship of this incident with his allegation of two sets of medical records. He ruled there was no obvious connection between the two unless the attorney could give a definite quote from the transcript. The plaintiff attorney thumbed through the transcript for three or four minutes, obviously not having marked the text where the cross-examination had occurred. Finally, his patience spent, the presiding judge severely lectured the attorney and ruled that this line of questioning would not be permitted any longer, that the cross-examiner had not made his point and had no evidence, and that he would not tolerate unwarranted attacks on the character of professional witnesses or any other witness without adequate proof. He apologized to the jury for having permitted an attack on the witness without facts and advised them to ignore the previous questioning.

There was clear liability in his case, but the plaintiff received a verdict of only three hundred and fifty dollars. Unquestionably, the jury reacted unfavorably to the obviously planned attack on a well-known, reputable physician, and had brought in what amounted to a defendant's verdict. It was apparent that the plaintiff's attorney in Smithville had forwarded a transcript of the previous trial to the other attorney, in another state, in an effort to discredit the expert witness and detract from his testimony, which he felt had damaged his own particular case and had resulted in a smaller award. It was also apparent that the Smithville attorney was so vindictive that he had gone to extraordinary limits to attack the defendant's witness.

Many of the lawyers engaged in negligence law in each jurisdiction are known to each other and are friendly competitors. Although they may attack each other in the courtroom, they are frequently observed having lunch together during the noon recess. In court it's a business problem, but outside they remain friends. There are few lawyers like the preceding one from Smithville who will go to any extreme to harass a medical expert whom he dislikes or fears. This particular attorney was very clever as well as disagreeable—and as it later developed, very persistent.

The orthopaedist had another encounter with him one year after his previous unpleasant experience. The defendant witness again appeared in Smithville as a defendant expert in another case tried by the same plaintiff attorney. This was an unusual case involving aseptic necrosis of the carpal navicular bone without fracture: there was considerable obscurity as to the origin of the lesion. The plaintiff, a young college professor, had sprained his right wrist too weeks prior to the auto accident under litigation, in which he suffered injuries to his shoulder and back. X-rays had been taken of his shoulder and back on the day of the accident, but he did not complain of pain in his right wrist until two weeks later. The past medical history revealed Legg-Perthes disease in childhood. One year after the car accident he developed Freiberg's infraction of the third metatarsal in his left foot, which had required surgery. All three of these conditions have a common denominator of aseptic or avascular necrosis, but there is no known report of a clinical entity of three such lesions in one individual.

The defendant witness testified that the avascular necrosis of the right wrist could have resulted from injury to the patient's wrist which occurred two weeks before the accident while repairing his car, but it also could be related to the other two incidents of avascular necrosis as a constitutional disorder. It was pointed out that had the patient injured his right wrist in the auto accident, after an injury to the same wrist two weeks previously early pain and disability would be anticipated; he would have complained of his wrist as well as of his upper back and shoulder. The witness further testified that it was not possible to relate the avascular necrosis of the wrist to the car accident with any probable degree of medical certainty, as the etiology could also have been the result of the previous accident or a pre-existing constitutional disorder. He further stated it was *possible* the auto accident could have aggravated the condition, but it was impossible to state the *probable* cause.

The cross-examining attorney, the doctor's previous adversary whom he had not seen since the other case, immediately proceeded to attack him to such an extent that the presiding judge intervened and pointed out that the doctor was not the defendant but only a witness. In his attack on the integrity of the defendant's witness, the plaintiff's attorney quoted the trial of his legal friend in the other jurisdiction to whom he had loaned the transcript of his own previous Smithville trial. It was quite obvious that they had exchanged files and transcripts and were teaming up to discredit the well-known defendant orthopaedist. The attack went something like this:

Q. Doctor, is it not true that you perform a great number of defendant examinations?

A. I do perform a significant number of such examinations, but I examine and treat many more plaintiffs than defendants.

Q. Obviously, you are testifying more often for the defendant than the plaintiff?

A. Yes, because I am usually called upon to examine only the more difficult defendant cases, those which are likely to go to trial. In addition, most of the plaintiff cases which I treat recover quickly in response to proper medical care; most of them are released within one month. Very few of these come to trial as the impartiality of the reports and fairness of the bills facilitate settlement in most cases.

Q. How many defendant exams do you perform in a week?

A. Perhaps 12 to 15 defendant cases, but I also examine and treat 35 or so plaintiff cases in a week.

Q. Isn't it true that when you testified in the case in Fairfield you stated that you examined 15 to 20 defendant cases a week, and 45 to 50 plaintiff cases a week?

This was an obvious attempt to show that the doctor was inconsistent in his testimony, as the variation was small and not significant. The witness replied that the previous testimony related to his practice in August, in which month a greater number of orthopaedists are away on vacation and his practice load increases; also that the nature of his practice varies from month to month because of many factors, such as emergency room coverage in several hospitals which brings many accident cases into his office. He added that he had answered the cross-examiner's question by analyzing his practice of the previous week.

The above questioning appeared to be a weak effort to demonstrate inconsistency in the doctor's testimony, as the number and type of cases seen varies from week to week and cannot be accurately stated without referral to office records.

The cross-examiner next asked for the doctor's clinical file on the case and after careful review, found nothing of significance.

He then quoted from another monograph in which the witness had written: "Before coming to trial the physician should review his records and remove any material that may prove embarrassing." This was quoted to the physician because the cross-examiner found nothing embarrassing in the file. In response the witness stated that this referred to correspondence with the referring attorney, perhaps written by the attorney himself, relating to fees, possible court appearance, or the attorney's own impression of the patient and the case, none of which were pertinent to the medical factors or his opinion. The doctor then asked the cross-examiner to read the next sentence in the monograph, which said, "This pertains to correspondence between the attorney and the physician, ...," just as he had answered. (The doctor had been asked this question before and remembered the paragraph very well.) Obviously this challenge had backfired on the cross-examiner, who then began a more vicious attack on credibility, again questioning whether he kept two sets of records, etc.

The judge again intervened and advised the attorney that the doctor was not a defendant, only a witness. The attorney then requested permission to approach the bench, where he indignantly pointed out that the rulings were very injurious to his client's case and the jury would get the impression that the judge was trying to protect the doctor. He was strongly advised by the judge that he would protect *any* witness, a professional witness or a lay witness, against unfair attack without absolute evidence to the contrary.

There was no rule on witnesses and the plaintiff's orthopaedist was in the courtroom during the previous exchange of testimony. The defendant orthopaedist had been taken out of turn, as the plaintiff's physician was from a distant city and did not arrive on time. The other orthopaedist was familiar with the reputation of the defendant's witness and may have resented the vicious, unwarranted attack on another physician. His testimony was considerably weaker than his written report, and he agreed that it was impossible to state with any degree of medical certainty that the accident had caused the avascular necrosis of the wrist. The plaintiff's orthopaedist may also have been influenced by the testimony he heard from the defendant's orthopaedist, which followed established medical knowledge. Because the treating orthopaedist could not establish a definite causal relationship between the injury and the accident, the court ruled in favor of a motion for a defendant's verdict, and the case did not go to the jury.

OBSERVATION OF OPPOSING ATTORNEY

When the doctor is testifying as an expert for the plaintiff or defense, it is wise to look at the opposing attorney and to observe him when he scribbles memoranda during his direct testimony, as such notes are usually made as a basis for questions to be asked during his cross-examination. By such observations the doctor will be better prepared for the cross-examination, and he can anticipate the subject of the questions. However, it is also possible the attorney plans to use these notes when he questions his own witness later in the trial.

An example of such observation was demonstrated in an out-of-town trial in which the orthopaedist testifying for the defendant noted with surprise that the plaintiff's attorney was making notes during the recital of his medical background which qualified him as an expert. Inasmuch as this is usually routine and both attorneys were familiar with the witness, the doctor speculated that there would be cross-examination on one particular point, noting that the attorney had scribbled a note as he was recounting his various medical papers. The doctor was not disappointed: the attorney did question him about his publications just as he had anticipated. He was asked about a monograph dealing with medico-legal medicine and widely distributed in pamphlet form. The witness realized that the attorney intended to discredit his testimony by demonstrating that he was a *professional* witness, who even taught other doctors how to testify.

However, as we found in the section on "qualifications," this point boomeranged as the doctor courteously replied that this particular pamphlet had been prepared as a hand-out at a scientific exhibit sponsored by the American Academy of Orthopaedic Surgeons at its annual convention. In response to a question regarding its contents, he stated that a principal aim was to improve reports prepared by orthopaedists in medico-legal cases, and also to upgrade their testimony, in order to facilitate the resolution of lawsuits involving personal injuries. As the witness was leaving the stand, the judge asked if he would send him a copy of the pamphlet for his own use. Obviously this must have impressed the jury and may have increased the weight of the doctor's testimony. A minimal verdict for the plaintiff was returned by the jury despite clear liability; the verdict was inadequate to cover his medical expenses and witness fees.

MISQUOTES

In his cross-examination the opposing attorney may try to trick the defendant's expert by misquoting his direct testimony or his statistics in order to discredit or depreciate his evidence. The medical witness may be asked such questions as what proportion of his practice is delegated to examination of defendants, how often he testifies in such cases, and what proportion of his income is derived from those sources. If defendant examinations represent a major portion of his practice, this could influence the jury by indicating possible prejudice toward a doctor who depends upon insurance companies for a substantial part of his income.

In response to such questions the doctor may reply that i.e., five to ten per cent of his practice consists of defendant examinations for various attorneys and companies (he should never use the word "insurance"!). Later the attorney may ask another question in which he falsely indicates ten to twenty as the percentage of the physician's defendant practice. The doctor should immediately point out the discrepancy and correct the attorney, as otherwise the latter will note in his summary that no exception was taken. He will use the larger figures to indicate to the jury that the doctor had a substantially greater interest in defendant examinations than he had originally testified.

An example was observed in a case in Alexandria, Virginia,

where the doctor testified under cross-examination that 5 to 10 per cent of his practice consisted of defendant examinations. In rephrasing the question, the plaintiff attorney slyly indicated 10 to 15 per cent, but the doctor corrected it. Later the doctor stated he examined approximately 10 to 15 *defendants* a week, but the cross-examiner indicated 15 to 20 in a following question; again he was corrected. A few moments later, the doctor testified he examined and treated 40 to 50 injured plaintiffs per week, but in a following question the cross-examiner lowered this to 30 to 40. These repeated misquotes represented an obvious attempt to impugn the impartiality of the testifying physician.

The above incident emphasizes that the physician should always be on the alert for any misquotation of his testimony; even though the apparent *error* appears inconsequential, he should always correct the attorney and again state the facts as he had previously testified. The jury will respect the witness who insists on correct factual information, and his evidence will be more impressive.

ALLEGED INCONSISTENCIES IN MEDICAL REPORTS

Personal injury cases which receive extended care for several months or longer necessitate medical reports at periodic intervals. Follow-up reports are also sent to the attorney if the patient returns at a later date for re-evaluation or further treatment. The doctor should strive for consistency in reporting his medical findings, and explain any variations or changes in the patient's condition.

In recording objective features of his repeated examinations the physician may realize that apparent inconsistencies have no real significance because of variable factors. However, an opposing attorney may emphasize these minor details in an attempt to discredit the witness as inefficient and inconsistent. For example, the leg length measurements in an adult should be identical when measured a year apart, unless there has been an intervening injury. The physician may record equal leg lengths on each visit, but if he uses different tape measures for each examination, or places the tape at a slightly different point, the total length may vary from ¼ inch to ½ inch from his previously reported figures. An experienced physician will recognize that there may be a difference in the tension and flexibility of a tape measure, and also that he may place the tape measure close to the malleolus in one instance and not as close the next time. It is important that he adopt one technique and remain consistent.

In measuring comparative circumferences of the calves and thighs, the physician should use a consistent technique by measuring an equal distance from the malleolus to the maximum circumference of the calves and the lower thighs, using ink or a wax pencil to mark these points. If the measurement is made at a point ¼ to ½ inch higher on one calf than the other, the calf circumferences will vary. However, if equidistant points are used on both lower extremities for repeated evaluations, the difference between the two measurements will remain the same.

In the following case the patient was a plump middle-aged female who had incurred an undisplaced fracture of the lateral malleolus, which had caused varying degrees of recurrent swelling of her calf. At the trial her treating physician, who had a reputation as a frequent defendant witness, testified to the permanent disability of the plaintiff, and reported his measurements of her lower extremities from several examinations made over a two-year period. The defendant lawyer was familiar with the witness, who was regularly employed by his firm for defendant examinations and reports. Despite this relationship, which mostly involved his legal partners in the firm, the defense attorney began a detailed attack on the credibility of the witness, then deliberately prolonged his cross-examination as he knew that the doctor had surgery in the afternoon which would interfere with his return to court after the lunch recess.

The cross-examiner continued the testimony in great detail, charting every measurement and date on a blackboard so that they could be compared. It was obvious that he was trying to demonstrate repeated variations and inaccuracies in the figures; the witness explained that the differences were due to the use of different tape measures on each visit. The attorney derided the witness regarding the elasticity of steel tape measures and tried to create the impression that this was just a cover-up for inconsistency. After 45 minutes of cross-examination, the judge suddenly recessed for lunch; this caused consternation in the witness who informed the court that he was due in surgery in 45 minutes. But the judge told the witness in no uncertain terms that he must return after lunch and again take the witness stand. The witness realized that since he was still on the witness stand, he would be in contempt of court if he did not return. He had no choice but to cancel the surgery and reschedule it, necessitating inconvenience and unnecessary expense to the hospital, the patient, and his family.

Of course the defendant attorney had anticipated this situation and had harassed the witness in an attempt to force the witness to testify favorably, and thus be free to leave the courtroom as quickly as possible. During the luncheon recess the testifying doctor spoke with the plaintiff (his patient) and her attorney. The patient informed the doctor that her weight had varied considerably in the two-year period covered by his several medical examinations. It was recognized immediately that this factor could have caused variations in the total size of her legs, although the difference between both calves had persisted unchanged. The doctor went to his car where he happened to have two different tape measures, both steel but of different flexibility. He also suggested to the plaintiff's attorney that he ask a question regarding his commitment to testify the following day in another court for a member of the cross-examiner's legal firm.

Testimony resumed and the doctor stressed that the patient's weight had escalated up and down considerably in the past two years, and also demonstrated the two tape measures with differences in flexibility, both of which would account for variations in measurement. This incensed the opposing lawyer, and he then asked the doctor how the patient was referred to him; he was advised it was a referral from the plaintiff's attorney. Under redirect examination the doctor was asked if the defendant attorney had ever referred clients to his office. The doctor promptly pointed out that he had many referrals from the other attorney's office, and as a matter of fact he was to testify the following day as an expert for that very same firm. The defendant attorney reddened, rose to his feet and angrily asked if it were not his partners who had used his services and not himself! This evidence negated the defendant's attack on the doctor's credibility as a witness, as it was now clear that his own firm had regularly employed his services. Incidentally, the doctor was not invited to the defense counsel's annual Christmas Party the next month!

HARASSMENT BY A "FRIENDLY ATTORNEY"

The physician who is interested in medico-legal practice will have frequent contacts with both plaintiff and defendant attorneys and often develop pleasant friendships with these members of the legal profession. A cordial relationship with exchange of ideas is of mutual benefit and eases the burdens of practice.

However, this friendly atmosphere may be strained at times as most attorneys accept cases for both plaintiff's and defendants, and the physician may occasionally find himself on the opposite side. In actual practice legal firms that specialize in defense of personal injury claims receive few plaintiff cases, but this does vary considerably with each group of lawyers. Thus it is possible that a defendant expert may examine a patient on behalf of an insurance company, and later learn that the patient is being represented by an attorney whom he has previously known only as a defense counsel.

At trial the physician may be surprised to encounter his legal friend sitting in the courtroom on the side opposite from the one to which he is accustomed; he then realizes that after giving his testimony he will be cross-examined by the lawyer for whom he has given direct testimony on many occasions. The doctor must be understanding if the cross-examination is intensive or irritating, as each attorney is morally and ethically bound to perform his services on behalf of his client to the best of his ability. Occasionally, however, some attorneys go far beyond reasonable inquiry in an effort to secure a large recovery. In these instances apparently the tantalizing sight of *the green poultice* (money) strains the ties of friendship and previous business associations. These attorneys have a greater interest in the immediate monetary award than in good will in future professional relations with the witness.

The following case involved a physician who had examined many clients and had testified frequently for an attorney who specialized in defending against personal injury actions. The attorney was of good reputation, but some of it was derived from his father, who was a widely known barrister of high standing in the community. The doctor testified for the defense after having examined a plaintiff represented by this attorney. He realized that he would be cross-examined on his testimony but he did not anticipate the strong attack on his character by one he knew so well. The plaintiff's attorney made a personal attack, using one-half hour of cross-examination in an attempt to characterize the doctor as an experienced defendant witness who did a great deal of work for insurance companies and other defendants (including himself). He made obvious attempts to have the witness use the word *insurance,* which would have caused a mistrial. His entire cross-examination related to the character of the witness. At no time did he question the doctor on his medical evidence, which was consistent with the testimony of his own doctor except for the prognosis. He cross-examined the doctor at length in typical plaintiff fashion about his bill and the amount of time spent with the patient. The witness testified that the examination itself took 45 minutes, but this did not include review of records and travel time for a special appointment to examine the plaintiff at a hospital near his home as requested by the plaintiff, which of course caused a greater loss of time from his practice. He had charged seventy-five dollars for the consultation which involved a complete examination of the neck and back, plus twenty-five dollars for review of extensive records and an additional report. In his questioning the attorney claimed that one hundred dollars was an excessive fee for *45 minutes' time,* realizing full well that more than forty-five minutes was involved in the examination, the preparation of two medical reports, and travel to and from a hospital in another county.

The witness was first amazed, then incensed with this line of questioning, and in reply stated that the attorney was fully aware of the answers, as he had testified on his behalf on numerous occasions and was familiar with his fees, methods, and type of practice. On redirect examination he informed the jury that he had testified on the side of the plaintiff attorney many more times than for the attorney defending this particular case.

After the trial, the doctor concluded that he should not have any further business association with this attorney. After all, if he really believed that the doctor was a prejudiced witness who testified principally for insurance companies—a rather strange posture for him inasmuch as he represented many insurance companies—then his estimate of the doctor's capability must be quite low.

After having rejected his initial desire to write the attorney a strong letter, the physician adopted the wiser course of phoning him. The lawyer told the doctor that he had made the attack because the doctor had "characterized his client as a malingerer." The doctor informed him that he had never used the word at all, nor did he state anything to that effect in any of his testimony. The lawyer replied that it had been done in a "round-about way." The doctor had testified that the patient was exaggerating, but he did not state that this was willful malingering; he informed the attorney that had he asked a direct question regarding malingering, he would have answered in the negative. The attorney agreed that perhaps he had been wrong, and in the future it would be preferable to ask questions regarding medical testimony rather than make a personal attack on the witness. This answer did not adequately explain the lawyer's unprincipled and unwarranted assault on a medical expert who had served him well in previous cases of difficult litigation. However, it was apparent that the attorney was interested only in his immediate problem, and obviously lacked the perspective and good judgment to preserve further relationships with his medical experts. His decision to alter his method of cross-examining a professional expert of long acquaintance may have been affected by the jury verdict in this case—one thousand dollars for multiple injuries with uncontested liability. This was little more than the medical and hospital expenses.

This incident illustrates that personal attacks on a physician of good reputation with courtroom experience rarely benefits the aggressor attorney.

INSERTION OF EVIDENCE

A medical expert is not always given the opportunity to present all of his evidence during the direct examination by his own attorney. This may occur because of the rules of evidence which restrict his testimony (i.e. hearsay evidence or the fact that other witnesses have not yet testified and laid the foundation for his opinions, etc.), or because of his attorney's ineptness (forgetting to ask him pertinent questions). However, a clever witness is often able to insert additional information or opinions in response to a detailed cross-examination which probes into new aspects of the case which were closed until the opposing attorney asked the question which *opened the door.*

An alert attorney recognizes a formidable witness and frequently foregoes cross-examination, other than by a few innocuous questions, in order to prevent him from augmenting his testimony. Through his replies to the opposing lawyer, an expert witness is often able to emphasize salient points in his direct testimony, and also to clarify or rectify any obscure facts or opinions which he believes to be of significant value to the case. It is in the cross-examination phase of the trial that the expression, "Be careful not to open Pandora's box," applies most accurately. One ill-advised question may adversely affect the outcome of the trial. If the witness does not utilize the opportunity, it is quite likely that his attorney will recognize it and develop the new evidence during his re-direct examination of the medical expert.

A good example of this situation occurred during a trial in a Maryland Circuit Court a few years ago. The patient was an irresponsible painting contractor (so-called) who worked irregularly and obviously had some other source of income. He was involved in a minor automobile accident in which his car was struck from the rear, resulting in a cervical strain which required only minimal medical care. However, he continued to claim a persistent pain in his neck which interfered with his job as a journeyman painter. The defendant's examination was entirely negative and did not reveal any objective basis for his complaints. In addition to the medical reports involving the recent auto accident, the examiner was also provided with a hospital record of treatment for a fractured leg five years before; this related the manner in which the injury was sustained—by jumping out the third story of a building which was not on fire. There was an obvious question why a person would jump from the third story of an intact building; the pre-trial investigation had revealed a police raid. However, this evidence could not be reported in court as it had been ruled inadmissible.

In his direct testimony the defendant's orthopaedist had stated that he found it difficult to believe that the patient was having as much pain, disability and suffering as he alleged. He concluded that a great many of the patient's complaints were exaggerated. During the cross-examination the plaintiff attorney naïvely asked the orthopaedist why he was so sure that the patient was exaggerating. Did he have any basis for not believing the statements made to him by the patient? The orthopaedist first mentioned the lack of any positive clinical findings in his thorough examination, then quietly mentioned the history given him by the patient of having been treated five years before at the County Hospital for a fractured leg after jumping out a third-story window of a building which he confirmed was not on fire.

At this point the attorney objected on grounds that the medical record pertaining to that incident had been ruled inadmissible. However, the judge instructed the attorney that he himself had opened up the subject by asking his question, and the doctor now had a perfect right to answer. The doctor then briefly pointed out that the patient told him he had fallen out of a third story window when he broke his leg, whereas the hospital records clearly stated that he had *jumped* out the window. He also testified that the patient refused to clarify the discrepancy. This certainly impugned the credibility of the patient, as there were obviously undisclosed facts relating to this incident.

Although there was clear liability in this case, the patient was awarded only four hundred dollars for his medical expenses. Apparently the jury had correctly interpreted the evidence and concluded that this man was a professional gambler whose statements could not be accepted as truthful.

REACTION TO ABUSE

Under no circumstances should the testifying physician become rattled and angered by the attacks of a cross-examining attorney. Although most attorneys are gentlemen and treat their professional colleagues with respect according to the code of ethics of the American Bar Association, there are a few who are overly aggressive, abusive, and provocative in their attempts to break down the testimony of an opposing physician, particularly when he is testifying for the defendant. Such tactics often backfire by arousing the hostility of the court, particularly when the attack is unjustified and the physician is of established repute. The attorney will often try to attack the credibility of the witness by demonstrating that he has testified many times before for the defendant, and that he is a "defendant-type physician." The witness should remain calm and unflustered and answer questions fully, realizing that he is not bound to merely answer *yes* or *no* but may qualify his answers, even though the attorney may try to cut him off with a *yes* or *no* answer. The court usually rules that the physician may explain his reply. The physician should not be intimidated by these tactics, but should insist upon giving a full explanation of his *yes* or *no* initial response.

A good example was observed in a recent North Virginia case which involved an elderly female nurse, the wife of a retired physician, involved in a minor automobile accident. The patient's complaints were grossly exaggerated and she continued to complain after a long course of proper therapy. After the examination for the defendant, the patient had made an oft-heard claim that the doctor had hurt her during the examination; she stated that the doctor had been rough, and her condition was aggravated as a result of the defendant consultation, a claim frequently made by individuals with minimal injuries and exaggerated symptoms.

When examined the patient was wearing a foam rubber cervical collar, but she was wearing it in a reversed position with the narrow opening anteriorly instead of posteriorly; this permitted her to move her neck freely, particularly in forward flexion where the support is generally required after a neck injury. The patient told the defendant examiner that her physician had advised her to wear the collar in that manner. She also stated that since the accident one year before she only wore the collar for long automobile trips and at night (when the need would be minimal), and had not been using it regularly for some time; yet she wore it to the office that day. At the trial, a year after the defendant examination and two years after the accident, the patient appeared in court wearing the collar regularly during the several days of the proceedings, again in the wrong position.

As the patient sat in court at her attorney's side it was obvious to all that she moved her head and neck quite freely with little restriction. While on the witness stand the defendant physician pointed to the improper use of the collar which was easily apparent to the adjacent jury. He also observed that the patient had stated to him a year earlier that she had not been using the collar for some time, except under special circumstances. The irate plaintiff lawyer then arose and began a tirade against the physician, immediately attacking his credulity. His first question, "Is it not true that you perform *all* of the defendant examinations for the firm of Black and Jones?" The doctor answered that he did perform occasional examinations for that firm, but he doubted (as he had no access to their records) that he performed *all* of their examinations—the judge immediately sustained an objection by opposing counsel. The cross-examining attorney then continued in the same vein, pointing out several firms which employed the physician for defendant examinations. On redirect examination the defendant attorney elicited information from the witness that the last two times the doctor had testified for him were not in a defendant capacity but on behalf of plaintiffs whom he represented.

The cross-examiner then became vicious in his attacks, having been bitterly stung by the demonstrated inconsistency in the use of the collar and evidence of impartiality of the expert witness which resulted from his own cross-examination. He tried to elicit testimony that the reverse position of the collar could be considered proper use. He was advised that there is an adjustable plastic cervical collar used to treat cervical strains, but this has the adjustable feature in front to raise and support the chin, thus demonstrating the importance of the anterior support. Other types of cervical braces with turnbuckles are designed to give support under the chin and occiput. Traction is often applied with the neck flexed for maximum opening of the neural foramina. The defendant medical expert was the final witness, and shortly thereafter the jury brought in a defendant's verdict. After the trial several jurors revealed that their decision was strongly influenced by the poor credulity of the plaintiff and the abusive courtroom antics of her attorney. Another striking feature in the adverse evidence was the lack of any treatment until two months after the accident; yet the patient claimed great disability and pain during this initial period. It was pointed out by the defendant expert that, as a physician's wife, treatment was available to her without charge had she required it.

HELPFUL POINTERS FOR CROSS-EXAMINATION

The following pointers are addressed to the expert medical witness facing cross-examination in court:

1. Talk with sufficient volume so that your voice carries to the jury. Use simplified language and explain any technical terms, using your body to illustrate if necessary. Do not overemphasize replies to questions from the cross-examining attorney. Maintain the same poise and demeanor exhibited during your direct testimony. Answer with a simple *yes* or *no,* not with a belligerent *Never!,* or *Absolutely—no doubt about it!*

2. Answer questions directly and completely, but briefly. Feel free to refer to your notes if necessary. If you believe the question is unfair or that the attorney is badgering you, look at your counsel before answering; if he fails to object, then you may turn to the judge and ask whether you should answer the question.

3. Don't get angry—restrain your temper! Your losing it is what the cross-examiner wishes would happen—when you are angry, you become careless and may say things that you later will regret, and you may *open the door* for further undesirable questioning. Your image to the jury will also be diminished if you become angry or sarcastic.

4. Don't elaborate in your answer. You may use an opportunity to insert a positive point that you have omitted during your direct testimony, but be careful that you do not provoke a new line of questioning.

5. Try to anticipate the next question by the nature of the questions being asked. Frequently the attorney will ask apparently obvious and innocuous questions to lay the ground work for a dramatic question which would be helpful to his cause. Pause and think before you answer, for once you have made a statement it is difficult to backtrack. If you have reviewed the material with your own attorney prior to trial, you should be able to avoid such traps by giving the correct answers to his preliminary inquiries.

6. Do not be forced into giving a *yes-or-no* answer if you feel that it does not convey the whole truth; state that you cannot give a straightforward *yes-or-no* answer without qualifying it. If the attorney insists that you answer *yes* or *no*, you may request the judge for permission to qualify your answers; however, usually your own attorney will interpose an objection to secure a ruling for you.

7. When questioned about quotations from textbooks or periodicals, remember that the attorney will only read the portion that is favorable to *him*. If you are not familiar with the article, request to see the whole text before answering. Frequently, you will note a sentence or two before or after the quotation which qualifies the portion read and changes its entire context.

8. Be careful in recognizing authorities quoted by the opposing attorney. Avoid using superlatives in recognizing any so-called

authority, as the opposing attorney will probably capitalize on this point. Most important of all, remember that in this particular case you are an authority, as you have examined the patient and you have specific medical knowledge about him. What applies to many patients in general may not apply to this particular patient. If you are a certified specialist, your opinion is just as worthy in this particular case as any recognized medical authority. Do not be boastful, but on the other hand do not be too modest.

9. When asked to comment upon the competence of a colleague, avoid any derogatory remarks. If he is competent, say so but without superlatives. If you do not wish to make any statement, state that you have "no opinion." With this reply you may be able to evade an embarrassing question about another practitioner or statements which may lead to malpractice charges against him. When you state you have no opinion, there is nothing further that can be asked of you.

10. A frequent question on cross-examination by a plaintiff's attorney will be, "Doctor, how many times did you examine the patient?" followed by, "How long did you spend with the patient?" Usually a good answer is, "I spent enough time to make an adequate examination and write a detailed report. I don't keep a time record, so I do not have the exact time available; even if I did, it would not be accurate as I may have been interrupted by phone calls. Usually such an examination requires forty-five minutes to one and one-half hours (time mentioned depends on your routine); I do not charge according to time."

This question is obviously an attempt to harass and depreciate the medical expert. It is of dubious significance as the doctor may be able to make a diagnosis in a few seconds, such as stenosing tenosynovitis of the thumb, whereas in other cases considerable time is required for an accurate evaluation. If you wish, you may draw an analogy with the motor problems of your car; you may have spent a great deal of time going from mechanic to mechanic without finding out what was wrong with the car. Then you go to a carburetor specialist, and within a few minutes he finds the trouble and repairs it. The charge you make for professional services is for your knowledge, not simply the amount of time involved. The doctor should emphasize that it is not the amount of time that is spent with the patient that counts, but what is done with that time. Another example is a college student who may spend four years in college but leave college with little education and knowledge. Another individual will use his time much more wisely and expertly and in a lesser period of time emerge from college with more wisdom and better preparation for the future. The amount of time spent is not entirely relevant— it is *how* it is used that is important.

The doctor may also explain that a medical specialist is often called upon to make a diagnosis and decide upon a course of treatment in the initial consultation. After a specialist has examined a patient on one occasion at the office or hospital, he usually arrives at a diagnosis and recommends a course of treatment. Occasionally the medical expert may return after having ordered special laboratory tests and render his final decision at that time. It is routine for a medical school professor to render a definitive opinion in a complex medical problem presented to him for the first time on medical rounds with students or residents. The usual clinical consultation is one-half hour to one hour in duration, followed by a definite diagnosis which is usually adequate and satisfactory. Thus there is a long established precedent for a medical specialist to express an opinion after one visit of 30 to 60 minutes' duration.

The clever attorney will press the point by asking the doctor, "Did you take a history?" and then, "How much time was spent in taking the history?" This is done to show that very little time was actually spent in examining the patient. However, the history is a very important part of the examination, and may disclose the need of various tests for clarification and diagnosis.

The treating doctor may take care of a patient over a long period of time without improvement. The persistent complaints may be due to either a failure to recognize the true causes of his difficulty, or improper or inadequate medical care. In such cases it is common to request the aid of a medical expert. The consultant usually sees the patient once, and he is often able to correct the patient's problem by making the correct diagnosis or ordering the proper treatment. Thus, although he may only see the patient once, if he is a competent expert, he may do more good for the patient than the treating physician who has cared for the patient for many months. This would invalidate the hypothesis that assumes that a doctor who sees the patient many times is in a better position to evaluate his condition than an expert consultant who has had only one contact with that patient.

A defendant examination is usually very detailed and exact, incorporating many objective measurements and tests. By contrast a plaintiff's doctor only infrequently makes as thorough an examination, even though he may have seen the patient on numerous occasions. Consultants for the plaintiff often do not perform as thorough an examination or write as comprehensive a report as the defendant's consultant. Therefore the doctor may answer that although he only examined the patient for 45 minutes, his examination was more complete than that revealed by medical records of the patient's own doctors. He may be able to demonstrate this by a direct comparison of the plaintiff's report and his report, placing them side by side and showing what was incorporated in each report. Despite the fact that he may have seen the patient only once, he had probably done a more thorough examination than the doctor who saw the patient many times.

With regard to the number of visits, most patients expect to be told what is wrong with them on the initial visit to their doctor. It is not necessary to have a patient return on numerous occasions before reaching a conclusion concerning diagnosis and treatment. A competent and experienced physician can usually make a correct diagnosis on the first visit if all the facts are before him.

Now to go back to what provoked this piece of advice, the doctor should realize that the harassing line of questioning indicates an effort to deflate the defendant's testimony, and at the same time increase the value of the evidence set forth by the treating physician, as he has usually seen the patient many more times than the defendant examiner. The actual facts are well known to the cross-examiner: first, that it is often difficult to get patients to submit to even one defendant examination, sometimes requiring a court order when the patient or his attorney refuses to cooperate; second, that it is unusual to have the opportunity for another examination. This is another reason why x-rays should be taken freely, because usually there is no second opportunity. X-ray evidence will not only strengthen responses to cross-examination, but represent strong objective evidence which carries considerable weight for the court and jury.

It should also be pointed out that the consultant often has an advantage over the treating physician if he sees the patient at a later date, as he has available a compilation of the medical records, indicating the complaints, response to treatments, activities, and so on. This gives him a comprehensive record of the patient's condition and helps him to prepare an objective report, whereas the physician who has constant intimate contact with a patient may involuntarily sympathize with the patient's condition or may actually be prejudiced in his favor. The regular treating physician who had known the patient prior to that accident, may have overlooked salient points in the history or examination. The old adage "you cannot see the forest for the trees" may apply; an objective observer may pick up points which should have been just as evident to the physician in frequent contact with the patient, but which escaped his attention because he was not as observant as the expert asked to make a complete evaluation of the case.

Another realistic point is that the defendant examiner usually has only one opportunity for his examination, a fact which is well known to the questioning attorney but upon which he wishes to capitalize. Should the doctor answer that he would have liked to have had further opportunities to repeat his examination, then the attorney will try to indicate that he is not able to express a definite opinion at that time, as he did not have the opportunity to examine and observe the patient as completely as desired.

Another demonstration of the value of a single consultation is observed when a consultant is called to the hospital to decide whether or not surgery is necessary. The experienced physician must make his decision then, not after weeks of observation. This does not lessen the value of his opinion; in fact, his recommendation is often final.

Thus this argument is obviously fallacious, and represents only a legal maneuver in our adversary system of justice.

11. If asked questions regarding fees, be prepared to explain your statement for services rendered by exhibiting a properly itemized bill. If your bill is extraordinarily high, have precise information and sufficient records readily available to substantiate the charges made; submit evidence such as a large number of office or hospital visits, treatment of complications, lengthy visits, and so on. A frequent method of attack is to demonstrate that the doctor greatly inflated his bill, implying his opinions are not entirely trustworthy; of course this would lessen the value of his testimony.

If asked, do not hesitate to state that you are charging a fee for appearing in court. The jury realizes that you should be paid for your services, but avoid mention of specific fees (low-salaried jurors do not appreciate the substantial fee of an expert witness). If you must give a figure, you may give a range, i.e. from one hundred to one hundred and fifty dollars, depending on the time involved, then stop; do not justify it with an explanation as this puts you on the defensive. A good answer, when asked how much you are being paid to testify, would go something like this: "I am not being paid for my testimony but for my professional knowledge and training, time spent in review of the medical facts, my medical opinions, and the amount of time I am kept away from my practice." You may also state (if true) that you have not made any specific arrangements for your fee. Sometimes, in reply to questions regarding fees, a light-hearted answer given with a smile is quite effective on the jury. In answer to "How much are you being paid to testify here today?" you may state, "Well, sir, I expect to be paid for the amount of time I am away from my practice, and that really depends upon how long you keep me here!" This usually draws smiles and takes the sting out of the point that the cross-examiner is trying to make, that you are prejudiced in your testimony because you are being paid to give it; frequently he will then cease this line of questioning. If a fee problem arises during the cross-examination, the attorney who called you to court will have the opportunity to ask you additional questions in his re-direct examination in order to clarify the issues.

Occasionally a desperate cross-examiner who has read this book will quote parts of the preceding paragraph to the witness who has utilized it in his replies regarding fees. The doctor should reassure the jury that the "low-salaried" label didn't apply to "that particular group of influential citizens," and that he was only being paid for the time lost from his practice, not for the contents of his testimony.

12. If you are not sure of an answer, you may take a moment to reflect upon it by asking the court for permission; then consider all aspects of the question before answering it. This does not denote weakness but demonstrates that you are taking your testimony seriously and giving it sober consideration.

13. Never *poke fun* at a cross-examining attorney, despite his apparent ineptness and lack of medical information. There is nothing to be gained by trying to depreciate his ability to the jury —if he really is incompetent, it will be apparent to the court before the case is completed, without your remarks. If you irritate him enough, he may deliberately draw out his cross-examination and prolong your loss of time from your medical practice.

14. Do not be lulled into a feeling of false security by the ingratiating, easy-going tactics of the opposing attorney. He may ask a series of short questions to which you can only answer in the affirmative, then suddenly put in a *sixty-four dollar question* of great import to the case, and hope you continue your rhythm of *yes* replies. Sometimes the attorney will turn away, apparently having completed his inquiries, then turn around and ask "just one more question"—a very pertinent one! If the witness does not give the reply the cross-examiner desires, he may follow it with a barrage of additional questions. It is a temptation for the witness to terminate his testimony by answering affirmatively, especially

after a tedious period of prolonged cross-examination, but he should stand by his principles and answer with his best judgment, no matter what the consequences.

15. Watch for *double-questions,* and questions that include an assumption of facts which have not been proven. The answer to each part of the double question may be different; the witness should take care to emphasize this in his reply, and also state that the assumed facts are not necessarily true.

16. Remain alert while under cross-examination and pay attention to all remarks that precede the questions. Most attorneys are astute, have a good vocabulary, and are well-versed in the significance of slight variations in words; they often try to shade their meaning to help their case. When you recognize this, do not let it pass, but promptly clarify the phrases used to correspond with the facts. However, do not try to cross verbal swords with a clever cross-examiner. Remember this is an everyday situation for him, and he is far more equipped than you for such a confrontation.

17. Be cautious in your answers when the cross-examiner asks you to confirm that "medicine is not an exact science." He is usually leading up to an admission that your medical opinion involves a significant degree of speculation or guesswork, thus decreasing the value of your previous testimony. Under the prevailing rules of evidence you are not required to be absolutely certain of your opinion, but only to a reasonable degree of medical certainty. Thus you should unequivocally deny that you have based your statements on speculation.

18. Don't over-react to the browbeating type of lawyer who badgers the witness and, approaching him, shouts questions and shakes his finger almost under the witness' nose. *Keep your cool,* as the current expression has it, turn to the judge, and quietly request that the attorney lower his voice and step back so that you may address your replies to the jury. The judge will also have become annoyed by these *assault tactics* and usually wel-

comes the chance to restrain a lawyer who is making a circus out of his dignified legal chambers.

19. Prolonged cross-examination can be exasperating, especially when it is obvious that the lawyer is tediously and deliberately prolonging your stay on the witness stand. This is apparent to the judge as well, but under our system of law he cannot intervene or direct the lawyer to stop, other than to inquire how much more time he will need to complete his inquiry so that he may set a time for recess. The lawyer knows that the doctor is anxious to return to his medical practice, especially if his testimony has been inserted into the proceedings out of turn in order to facilitate his busy schedule. The attorney may take advantage of the physician's harried position and prolong his examination in an effort to obtain favorable replies, probably counting on the doctor's hope of being excused shortly thereafter.

The medical expert should remember that when this occurs, it signifies that he has been an effective witness against the opposing counsel, and the prolongation is a desperate effort to break down his testimony.

Horsley sums up court proceedings with an apt quotation from John Quincy Adams: "Law logic is defined as an artificial system of reasoning, exclusively used in courts of justice, but good for nothing anywhere else!"[22]

9 USEFUL LEGAL FORMS AND PRINTED INSTRUCTIONS

Medical malpractice claims have become much more frequent in the past few years. Although many of them are without foundation, the doctor should employ all available means to avoid harassment from such suits. The doctor can no longer rely upon the mutual trust between patient and doctor which was so evident in past generations. Today he must have legal permission for many of his professional actions.

Many surgeons take photographs of patients, such as before and after plastic surgery or correction of severe orthopaedic deformities. Should the physician wish to use this later in the publication of a scientific article, legal permission of his patient is required.

Treatment of a minor requires consent of parents or legal guardian except in an emergency when immediate treatment is imperative and delay involves serious risk to the patient. Informed consent prior to surgery must be legally valid with an understanding of what is to be done and the risks involved. Consent for surgery for cosmetic purposes is a particularly vulnerable point for the plastic surgeon; consent must also be obtained for removal of tissue for grafting, as well as for sterilization, abortion, disposal of an amputated part, removal of an organ, radiation therapy, shock therapy in mental problems, use of radioisotopes, and agreement for blood transfusion—*all of these* require a valid written consent.

Physicians who undertake a clinical investigation with a new drug or use an experimental procedure or treatment must be particularly careful to obtain prior approval from the patients involved in the study. This represents a significant handicap in conducting the so-called *double blind* investigation, as the patient who signs a consent form must be informed that he may receive a placebo instead of true medication; this may not only reduce the number of patients who will consent to participation in the study, but also obscure the results.

For these and other such problems, a booklet outlining proper forms and legal analysis of same has been prepared by the legal department of the American Medical Association, and is available at a nominal cost. Every doctor should be familiar with this booklet and use the forms where indicated.[26]

Examples of forms and *hand-outs* to patients which should facilitate both medico-legal and clinical practice have been given. They may be reproduced without permission.

A form instructing the patient—for example, in after-cast care —provides the patient with complete instructions for observation of complications, very important after application of a cast. Pertinent exercises while in the cast can also be outlined on the same form. A notation should be made on the patient's chart that he has been given an instruction sheet; this affords the doctor protection from a malpractice claim that no instructions were received. Utilization of a written form not only insures that the patient has the instructions clearly and without misunderstanding, but it also saves the physician time.

The doctor should utilize any type of pre-fabricated form that is feasible for recording results of his history-taking, physical examination, and diagnosis. Some orthopaedists and neurosurgeons, who examine and treat a large number of personal injury cases, have devised elaborate and detailed forms of several pages to record this information in the shortest possible time. The author has found that dictating equipment in each examining room accomplishes the same purpose with more individual detail. However, this does have the disadvantage of the patient listening to the data recorded in his presence, whereas notations on printed forms afford more privacy. This particular factor is of more importance in the evaluation of defendants than plaintiffs. For this reason a basic examination form for an essentially negative examination of the neck, low back, lower extremities, eyes, ears, throat, heart and lungs has been devised; measurement data and additional findings can be inserted as indicated for each individual case.

Outlines of progress reports and final examinations pertaining to treatment of injuries of the cervical and lumbar spine are also suggested. It is anticipated that most physicians will modify these forms according to their individual examining techniques and mode of expression.

The treatment of musculo-skeletal injuries involves home care and exercise programs to achieve the best result as quickly as possible. It is essential that the patient be properly instructed in all phases of his home program. Printed forms with specific instructions eliminate misunderstandings and poor memory as an excuse for lack of cooperation. Although a brief oral explanation may still be necessary, written memoranda reduce the time required for treatment and discussion with the patient. Several such forms are freely distributed by pharmaceutical firms and others may be composed by the physician in accordance with his plan of treatment. Examples are printed in this text, but each physician may wish to devise his own forms according to his type of practice.

Many hospital emergency rooms give their out patients written instructions for follow up care, and require a signature acknowledging receipt.

10 CONCLUSION

AFTER WITNESSING SEVERAL COURTROOM EPISODES IN WHICH THE PHYSICIAN WAS EITHER GROSSLY UNPREPARED TO GIVE PROPER TESTIMONY OR HAD NO BASIC CONCEPTS OF LEGAL PROCESS, THE AUTHOR CONCLUDED THAT THERE WAS A POSITIVE NEED FOR INSTRUCTION AND EDUCATION OF MEDICAL WITNESSES. NUMEROUS ARTICLES AND MONOGRAPHS HAVE BEEN PREPARED FOR THIS PURPOSE, BUT MOSTLY BY ATTORNEYS WHOSE VIEWPOINTS, MOTIVATIONS, AND OBJECTIVES DIFFER FROM THOSE OF A MEDICAL CLINICIAN.

This book was written by a practicing physician to aid the doctor in his management of personal injury cases which involve litigation. The author's practice includes both plaintiffs and defendants; although the aim was to present the material in an impartial manner, it is apparent that his experiences as a defendant examiner and witness are predominant, and color some of his opinions and conclusions. The role of a fair and unbiased medical witness is much simpler and requires less medico-legal expertise than a defendant expert; he is also less apt to be challenged and abused by courtroom tactics.

The material presented is not comprehensive nor does it encompass every facet of medico-legal practice, as many texts have been written pertaining to specific aspects of forensic medicine, such as medical testimony, malpractice problems, suggestions to improve the doctor's court appearances, and collection of his fees. Many of these articles or books relate interesting courtroom experiences and impressions of courts, lawyers, and juries, but there appears to be need for a text which relates actual clinical experiences, to serve as a practical guide for both physicians and attorneys in medico-legal practice. This should lead to further

318

cooperation between the two esteemed professions and result in mutual benefit for all parties.

The title of this book indicates there are two professions involved in the resolution of litigation resulting from personal injuries. If these professions, medicine and law, can work together in a harmonious and cooperative manner, the matters under litigation can be settled fairly and amicably with mutual benefit to all concerned.

Some of the courtroom episodes recounted in this publication reflect harsh, acrimonious attacks in the cross-examination of competent medical experts, solely for the purpose of monetary gain. Although the attorney does have an obligation to his client, most jurists and lawyers believe this duty can be performed without resorting to unfair, harsh courtroom tactics and discourtesies to professional colleagues.

Several jurisdictions have prepared manuals to establish standards of conduct for the medical and legal professions, in order to promote harmonious relationships between attorneys and physicians. Although these codes are not binding upon individuals, they do establish a pattern of approved conduct to which the members of both professions are expected to adhere. With such cooperation many of the problems involved in the submission of medico-legal reports and in the appearance of medical witnesses for testimony should be greatly diminished.

The attached code of cooperation for Maryland physicians and attorneys, written by a joint committee from the bar and from medical societies, represents a model of inter-professional cooperation and respect. Extension of such a code to other communities will promote firm bonds of friendship and mutual respect for lawyers and physicians.

MEDICO-LEGAL CODE OF COOPERATION—MARYLAND

Preamble

Acknowledging that substantial part of the practice of law and medicine is concerned with the problems of persons who are in need of the combined services of a lawyer and a physician; that the public interest and individual problems in these circumstances are best served only as a result of cooperative efforts of all concerned;

that members of both the legal and medical professions share an obligation to the individual and to society, we the members of the Prince George's County Bar Association and the Prince George's County Medical Society, do adopt and recommend the following declaration of principles as standards of conduct for attorneys and physicians, in interrelated practice.

MEDICAL EXAMINATIONS AND REPORTS

1. **Authorization of Patient Required:** A physician shall furnish to any person, any information concerning the history, physical condition, diagnosis or prognosis of the physician's patient only upon the signed authorization of the patient (or, in the case of a minor, of the minor's parent or guardian, or where authorized by law.*

2. **Reports to Patient or his Attorney:** The patient, or his attorney, shall be entitled upon written request, to a prompt report from the attending physician, concerning the history, findings, treatment rendered, diagnosis and prognosis. The physician's fee for such report should be commensurate with the time and effort devoted to its preparation.

3. **Request for Report:** When a medical report is requested of a physician, whether he be an attending physician, consulting physician, or examining physician, the lawyer requesting the report should make clear in his request the specific information desired; should disability evaluation and the prognosis be desired, the lawyer should so specify.

4. **Examination of Adverse Party:** Where there has been an adverse party, the examining physician shall not furnish to the person examined or his attorney or anyone else other than the person arranging for the examination a copy of his report or any information concerning his findings on such examination. The examining physician, acting for a party adverse to the person he is examining, should, where taking a medical history, attempt to elicit only such facts as are pertinent to his examination.

MEDICAL TESTIMONY

1. **Conference Before Trial:** In order that the patient and client may have his case properly presented to the court or other tribunal and to see that justice is done, it is the duty of each profession to present fairly and adequately the medical evidence in legal controversies. To arrive at that end pre-trial conference between the

*Examinations made in Workmen's Compensation cases fall in this category.

lawyer and the physician regarding medical testimony is encouraged and recommended. The members of each profession shall do their utmost to cooperate with the other in arranging a time and place satisfactory to both for such a meeting.

2. **Subpoena for Physician: Conference:** A subpoena should not be issued to any physician without prior notice and conference with such physician, where possible, concerning the matters regarding which he is to be interrogated, unless the physician and the lawyer agree that such conference is unnecessary.*

3. **Cooperation with Court:** It is recognized that the proper and efficient dispatch of the business of the courts cannot depend upon the convenience of litigants, the lawyers or the witnesses, including physicians who may be called to testify; both the lawyer and the physician should recognize, accept and discharge their obligation to aid and cooperate with the courts in the presentation of medical testimony.

4. **Arrangement for Court Appearance:** In arranging for the attendance of a physician at a trial or other legal proceeding, the lawyer should always have due regard and consideration for the professional demands upon the physician's time, and accordingly, the lawyer should, whenever possible, give the physician reasonable notice in advance of his intention to call the physician as a witness, and of the probable date on which the physician will be expected to testify.† The lawyer should also advise the physician to bring with him to court such records as the lawyer or the physician may need for the proper presentation of the physician's testimony. Furthermore, during the course of the trial the lawyer should endeavor to keep the physician advised from time to time as to the approximate hour when he will be called to the witness stand; and upon the physician's appearance at the hearing at the hour agreed upon, the lawyer should endeavor to arrange with the court for the prompt calling of the physician to the witness stand.

When arrangements are later cancelled for the court appearance and the physician has cancelled his regular appointments, he shall, nevertheless, be entitled to be paid a reasonable fee.

5. **Fees for Expert Testimony:** A reasonable expert witness fee is a proper and necessary item of expense in litigation involving

*Careful preparation of a case requires that the lawyer issue a subpoena for each important witness including physicians. A lawyer should explain to the physician that the issuance of a subpoena for the physician is in accordance with the standard practice of procuring physicians as witnesses.

† It must be understood that the lawyer does not control the date of trail in any case since this is a matter in the sole control of the court.

medical questions. When a physician is called to testify as an expert witness, he should be paid such expert witness fee as may be agreed upon between the physician and the lawyer calling him. In every instance in which the lawyer makes arrangements for expert testimony it shall be the duty of the lawyer to see that the physician is paid his fee.

6. **Contingent Fees:** Neither the physician called as a witness nor the lawyer so calling him shall invite or enter into any arrangement whereby the making of a charge for the physician's appearance as a witness or for the giving of testimony, or the amount of any such charge, shall be contingent on the outcome of the litigation or on the amount of damages awarded in the case.

7. **Physician Called as Witness:** The attorney and the physician should treat one another with dignity and respect in the courtroom. The physician should testify solely as to the medical facts in the case and should frankly state his medical opinion. He should never be an advocate and should realize that his testimony is intended to enlighten rather than to impress or prejudice the court or the jury.

It is improper for the attorney to abuse a medical witness or to seek to influence his medical opinion. Established rules of evidence afford ample opportunity to test the qualifications, competence and credibility of a medical witness, and it is always improper and unnecessary for the attorney to embarrass or harass the physician.

PAYMENT FOF MEDICAL SERVICES RENDERED

Upon final disposition of any case wherein services rendered by a physician are involved, the lawyer shall forthwith notify the physician of such disposition and upon the receipt of the physician's bill and an order from the patient to pay the same direct to the physician, the attorney shall use every reasonable effort to see that the physician's bill is paid forthwith. The attorney shall make no charge to the physician for any services rendered in connection therewith. Unless otherwise agreed, the primary responsibility for payment of medical expenses rests with the client-patient.

COMMITTEE ON INTERPROFESSIONAL RELATIONSHIPS

For many years the Prince George's County Medical Society and the Prince George's County Bar Association, recognizing the need of a committee composed of both physicians and lawyers for the purpose of promoting a closer and more harmonious relationship between the two professions, have designated annually a group of physicians to work with a corresponding number of lawyers, the size of the committees to be within the discretion of each association. It shall consider all matters concerning interprofessional relationships between these two professions, including but not limited to the following:

1. Promotion and perpetuation of harmony between the professions.

2. Achieving a fuller understanding of mutual problems.

3. Consideration of legislation affecting medical-legal professional relationships.

4. Hearing of grievances stemming from interprofessional relationships.

5. Referral of grievances to the Medical Society or the Bar Association concerned where that committee deems such reference warranted.

PHYSICIAN/PATIENT RELATIONSHIP

The legal profession recognizes that the practice of medicine is a hazardous task and that it is obviously not always possible for the physician to obtain a good result even with the best of attention and professional skill, and that an unfortunate result does not indicate in itself that the physician did not exercise the highest degree of skill and attention in the treatment of the case; and that a lawyer should not undertake to make any claim against a physician without thoroughly investigating the essential facts and details and being reasonably certain that if a harm has been done a patient, that it was due to genuine carelessness or negligence or lack of professional skill as distinguished from honest difference of opinion or the difference in honest judgment in a particular case. It should, nevertheless, also be considered that by the Canons of Professional Ethics the lawyer owes devotion to the interests of his client, warm zeal in the maintenance and defense of his rights, and the exertion of his utmost learning and ability, and that the client is entitled to the benefit of any and every remedy and defense that is authorized by law, and he may expect his lawyer to exert every such remedy or defense that is authorized by law.

The medical profession recognizes that there are cases in which the patient suffers injury as a result of negligence, carelessness, or lack of professional skill on the part of a physician and that in these cases, there should be just compensation to the injured person. That in cases of this character, it is as much the duty of a physician-expert to assist the injured person as it is the duty of a physician-expert to defend a fellow-physician when he is proceeded against improperly.

GENERAL PROVISIONS

Nothing contained in this Statement of Principles is intended to be inconsistent with the rules of law, Canons of Ethics of the local, state and national Bar Associations and the Principles of Medical Ethics of the American Medical Association.

Although the Maryland Medico-Legal Code of Cooperation is considered to be an exemplary document in the promotion of better relations between the medical and legal professions, it has not received universal support from the Prince George's County physicians. An objection was made by a prominent orthopaedist to the furnishing of medical reports to lawyers in return for a countersigned assignment form. This orthopaedist has a firm rule that no reports are sent until the account has been fully paid. This is an acceptable procedure which has been adopted by some physicians, usually after adverse experiences in collection of their bill after settlement of the case; it is considered proper ethical practice. However, many patients are unable to pay their account in full prior to settlement of their claim, and in these instances the assignment plan is an effective method of management.

One physician, in discussing the code before the medical group, made the statement, "All lawyers are crooks." Several doctors objected to such a broad label for an honored profession, but this does represent an attitude which was formerly quite prevalent among doctors, although certainly unwarranted. Of course there are dishonest lawyers, but there are also dishonest members of every profession, including that of medicine. The *modus operandi* of a few attorneys have engendered this undesirable attitude but it obviously should not be broadened to include the entire profession. This is the type of situation that the Code attempts to overcome.

The increasing importance of the physician's participation and exposure to medico-legal matters has led to the formation of a separate organization devoted exclusively to this subject, The American College of Legal Medicine. The organization is composed principally of individuals who have degrees in both the medical and legal professions, but members of either profession may join the organization as an associate.

There are several professional journals, edited by both lawyers and doctors, which are devoted exclusively to medico-legal medicine. Increasing numbers of articles dealing with personal injury litigation are appearing in professional medical journals oriented toward economic and administrative problems in the practice of medicine.

———

Medico-legal examinations and reports present a real challenge to the interested physician; an accurate evaluation and presentation of medical data requires excellent diagnostic acumen, keen observation and perception, alertness and intuitiveness, and familiarity with many facets of medicine. "There is no substitute for experience," but ordinary common sense is also essential to a successful medico-legal practice.

In most cases involving patients the diagnosis and prognosis can be determined without question, but when elements of anxiety and nervous disorder, exaggeration, or malingering for monetary gain enter into the clinical picture, the physician must exercise his mental faculties and his sensitivity and intuition to the utmost in order to penetrate to the basic facts in a medico-legal problem. In most cases he will succeed in its solution, but even the most astute and experienced examiner will occasionally have some doubt as to one or another of his final conclusions.

The difficulties are more intense when a strong nervous element obscures residuals of organic injuries from injuries sustained during and in the aftermath of an accident; there may be considerable difficulty in identifying or separating one from the other. Experience has indicated that such problems occur most frequently with herniated lumbar disc or lumbar strain syndromes of long duration, which have not fully responded to either conservative or surgical treatment and have caused prolonged inactivity or disability with resultant economic loss. A vicious cycle develops as the nervous problem is aggravated by the enforced idleness from organic injury, which in turn predisposes the individual to over-concern and introspection because of his continued symptomatology and his apparent failure to respond to treatment. Injuries to other areas may also result in similar clinical patterns, such as cervical injuries with radicular pain to the upper extremities. All of these cases require the careful scrutiny of the physician who must also serve as expert witness in court.

A few physicians have the attitude that medico-legal cases are concerned only with financial gain and are therefore beneath the dignity of their particular practice. This is not based on the experience of physicians caring for large numbers of personal injury cases. Although there are such cases with built-up damages for greater compensation, most of these patients are honest citizens seeking a just recovery for personal damages, according to the prescribed laws and prevailing judicial practices of our country. However, they should receive only what is due them; it is the obligation of the treating and examining physician to indicate accurately and without exaggeration, how much damage resulted from the accident in litigation. He can achieve this purpose by taking a detailed medical history followed by a thorough medical examination and x-rays where indicated, then reaching a final conclusion and evaluation based on his experience and objective observations.

It is the author's belief that if these or similar methods are adopted by physicians caring for medico-legal cases, there will result a higher percentage of fair out-of-court settlements and a reduction in the large number of cases now filling our court calendars. In those cases which are actually litigated, the professional and fair testimony of an examining or treating physician will facilitate a just and fair verdict. This can be achieved if the physician gives these cases his careful, unprejudiced attention, and treats them in an objective manner.

BIBLIOGRAPHY

1. Aarons, Edward F.: Curing doctors' courtroom headaches. *Medical Economics,* April 3, 1967, pp. 29-35.
2. Belli, Melvin: Is the M.D. expert witness bound to full disclosure? *Medical World News,* Nov. 3, 1967, pp. 58-59.
3. Bordenave, J. L.: Don't let lawyers push you around. *Medical Economics,* April 28, 1969, pp. 139-147.
4. Brown, Kent: Compensation for the medical witness. Medicolegal Symposium, Miami Beach, Fla., March 1967.

5. Cattell, H. F. and Filtzer, David L.: Pseudo subluxations and their normal variations in the cervical spine in children. *Journal of Bone and Joint Surgery, 47-A*:1295-1309, Oct. 1965.

6. English, O. Spurgeon: How to recognize a psychosomatic case. *Hospital Medicine,* Sept. 1964, p. 29.

7. Enelow, Allen J.: Psychological factors of compensable injury. *Medical Tribune,* Oct. 31, 1966, p. 23.

8. Fargo, Steven: National Medicolegal Symposium, Las Vegas, Nev., March 1965.

9. Fineman, Sol *et al:* The cervical spine: Transformation of a normal lordotic pattern into a linear pattern in the neutral posture. *Journal of Bone and Joint Surgery, 45*:1175-1183, Sept. 1963.

10. Florence, David W.: You, too, can collect fees from lawyers. *Medical Economics,* Jan. 19, 1970, pp. 133-142.

11. Frenkil, James: How to manage the malingering patient. *Medical Economics,* March 18, 1968, pp. 187-200.

12. Gordon, Everett J.: Medico-legal examinations, reports and testimony. Scientific Exhibit, American Academy of Orthopaedic Surgeons, Chicago, Ill., Jan. 1966.

13. Gordon, Everett J.: Diagnosis and treatment of acute low back disorders. Bulletin of the Sibley Medical Association, Washington, D. C., 7:21-30, 1964.

14. Gordon, Everett J.: Injuries of shoulder and upper arm trauma. Albany (N.Y.), Matthew Bender & Co., April 1960, Vol. 1, No. 6, pp. 31-110.

15. Gordon, Everett J.: Knee injuries: Ligaments, bursae and menisci, trauma. Albany (N.Y.), Matthew Bender & Co., Dec. 1960, Vol. 2, No. 4, pp. 3-51.

16. Gordon, Everett J.: Fractures and dislocations of spine and pelvis, trauma. Albany (N.Y.), Matthew Bender & Co., June 1962, Vol. 4, No. 1, pp. 5-99.

17. Gordon, Everett J.: Fractures, dislocations of thigh, knee and leg, trauma. Albany (N.Y.), Matthew Bender & Co., Aug. 1964, Vol. 6, No. 2.

18. Gordon, Everett J.: Diagnosis and treatment of acute low back disorders. *Industrial Medicine and Surgery* (Miami, Fla.), Vol. 37, No. 10, Oct. 1968.

19. Gordon, Everett J.: Medico-legal examinations: Reports and testimony. *Southern Medical Journal, 61*:10, 45-51, Oct. 1968.

20. Gordon, Everett J.: Diagnosis and treatment of acute low back disorders. Scientific Exhibit and Annual Meeting, AMA, Atlantic City, N. J., June 1963.

21. Hitzelberger, W. E. and Witten, R. M.: Abnormal myelogram in

asymptomatic patients. *Journal of Neurosurgery* (Chicago), *28*: 204-206, March 1969.

22. Horsley, Jack E.: Testifying? Back up your words with pictures. *Medical Economics,* Jan. 17, 1972, pp. 193-195; March 29, 1972, pp. 89-91; April 24, 1972, pp. 129-136.
23. Jamar Adjustable Dynamometer instruction sheet, Asinov Engineering Co. (1414 S Beverly Glen Blvd), Los Angeles, Calif.
24. Johl, J. H., Muller, S. M. and Roberts, G. W.: Roentgenographic variations in the normal cervical spine. *Radiology,* 78:591-597, 1962.
25. Kraus, Hans: *Backache—Stress and Tension.* New York, Simon & Schuster, 1965.
26. Medicolegal forms with legal analysis. Law Department, AMA, 1961.
27. Medicolegal Symposium, Proceedings American Bar Association— American Medical Association, Miami Beach, Fla., March 1967.
28. Norton, Edward J., Jr.: Why spend time on medico-legal reports. *Medical Economics,* June 12, 1967.
29. Orange County (Calif.) Medical Association. Guide for determining physician fees in medico-legal cases. *AMA News,* May 26, 1969.
30. Packard, B. Gibson: Orthopaedic detection of malingering. *Southern Medical Journal, 60:*1233, Nov. 1967.
31. Robitscher, Jonas: The doctor as an occasional witness. *Modern Medicine,* June 30, 1969, pp. 78-81.
32. Schutt, Charles H., and Dohan, F. Curtis: Neck Injury to Women in Auto Accidents. *JAMA 206:*12, 2689-2692, Dec. 16, 1968.
33. Stewart, William J.: Medicolegal Symposia, Miami Beach, Fla. March 1967.
34. Sullivan, Philip R.: Is this symptom functional? *JAMA, 185:*745, 1963.
35. Threadgill, Francis D.: Whiplash injury, end results in eight-eight cases. *Medical Annals of the District of Columbia,* 29:226-228, 1960.
36. Williams, Harold: Compulsory court attendance. Medicolegal Symposium, Miami Beach, Fla., March 1967.

ILLUSTRATIONS

MEDICO-LEGAL EXHIBIT

Page

Frontispiece ii

Fig. 1. History Sheet 15

Fig. 2. Examination Form for Notations of Measurement 32

Fig. 3. Hand and Arm Evaluation 39

Fig. 4. Jamar Dynamometer 40

Fig. 5. Measurement of Range of Motion of Cervical Spine 42-45

Fig. 6. Examination of Back 48, 49

Fig. 7. Examination of Back 51-59

Fig. 8. Fracture of Neck of Femur, not visible on initial X-Rays 65-67

Fig. 9. Traumatic Aggravation of Pre-existing Arthritis 69-74

Fig. 10. Physician Must Be Astute. Use all your faculties! 102

Fig. 11. Home Paraffin Baths 123

Fig. 12. Buck's Extension Traction 124

Fig. 13. To Help Ease Your Back Pain 128

Fig. 14. Exercises for Low Back Pain 130-131

Fig. 15. Surgery for Rupture of Shoulder Cuff 161, 162

Fig. 16. Surgical Correction of Non-Union of Fracture of Elbow with
         Vitallium Prosthesis 163-168

Fig. 17. An Impartial Medical Opinion Carries Weight 170

Fig. 18. Don't Pontificate—Give Testimony, not a Lecture 240

INDEX

Accidents
  consultation with
    attorney prior to
    medical attention, 109
American College of Legal
    Medicine, 3, 324
Anxiety States, 101
    (see nervous factors, 325)
Appointments,
  cancellation or "no-shows"
    by plaintiffs for defendant
    examinations, 225
Arthrocentesis of joints, 125
Arthritis,
  post-traumatic, 118
Assignment Forms, 200, 201, 202
Assignment,
  medical pay coverage
    of patient, 202
  responsibility of attorney
    to pay physician, 206, 207
Attorney,
  false information regard
    representation, 215, 216
  investigation in cases
    of dubious liability, 215
  screening of accident
    cases for, 215
  suggestion of diagnoses, 138, 139
  witness to defendant
    examination, 28
Avascular necrosis,
  multiple manifestations
    in single patient, 290

Back, low,
  examination, 47-64
  strain, manifestations of 62
Back, treatment of injuries of
    home program, 127, 128, 130, 131

Casts,

after-care instruction
    sheets for, 134, 316
Cervical spine,
  examination of, 42
    (see examination, cervical spine)
Claims,
  for injury or aggravation by de-
    fendant examination, 92, 303
Code, Medico-legal, 319
Competency, professional
    judgement of, 9, 258, 259, 307
Conference,
  pre-trial, 248
Consultations, 125
Contrast baths, 135
Cross-examination,
  adverse reaction on cross-
    examiner's own medical expert
    sitting in courtroom, 292, 293
  anticipation of questions, 282, 306
  apparent irrelevant material in
    physical examination, 261
  attack on integrity of defendant
    expert, 303
  attack on qualifications, 293
  attempts to defame witness, by
    demonstrating inconsistency with
    his writings and previous testimony
    —case reports, 286-293, 295
  attorney referral of patient, 297
  basis, 279
  bill of treating physician, 311
  brief responses, 305
  calm demeanor, 305
  combined efforts of plaintiff
    attorneys to defame witness
    by exchange of trial
    transcripts, 288-293
  comments on competence of
    colleagues, 307
  dangers with effective
    witnesses, 280

331

defamation by "friendly
  attorney", 299
deliberate prolongation to provoke
  favorable testimony from
  witness, 314
desire for further examinations
  by defendant expert,
  significance of, 310
double questions, 313
fees for testimony, 284, 285, 311
harassment by attorney who
  frequently employs witness'
  services, 298-300
harassment by extended questioning
  to interrupt witness's schedule, 297
honest answers, 283
inconsistency of medical
  expert, 291, 295
insertion of new evidence,
  (case report), 301-303
introduction of new evidence, 280
judges' reaction to vicious
  attack on medical expert, 289, 292
loss of temper, 306
measurement, inconsistencies of,
  295, 296
medical-legal exhibit
  and pamphlet, 294
medical reports, inconsistencies of,
  295
medicine as an art,
  not a science, 313
misquotes, deliberate, 294
  correction of, 294, 295
observation of cross-examination
  during direct testimony, 293
off-guard questions, 312
opening of "Pandora's box", 301
opening of previously forbidden
  subjects, 281, 301
over-reaction to abuse, 313
plaintiff's physician, 295-298
post-trial difficulties with attorney
  after vicious cross-examination,
  300-301
purpose, 279
quotations from textbooks, 306
recognition of authorities, 306

recognition of textbooks as
  authoritative, 283, 284
reduction of effects of exaggerated
  testimony, 281
restraint, criticism of
  inept cross-examining
  attorney, 312
revised opinions after presentation of
  undisclosed evidence, 281, 282
study and preparation for, 282, 283
testimony in other trials, 285
time required for defendant
  examinations, 307
value of one defendant examination
  vs. multiple examinations of
  treating physician, 308, 309
witness' publications, 285
yes or no answers, 306

Deposition, 269
  for harassment, 276-277
Deposition, by subpoena,
  attempt to secure expert opinions
    without due compensation, 271,
    272
  fees, 269, 270
  illustrative case, 271
  imposition requiring excessive
    travel, 270, 271
  place of, 269
  quashing for unreasonable
    demands, 278
  result of court action to compel
    expert testimony (illustrative
    case), 273-275
Diagnosis,
  anxiety states, 101
  attorney suggestions for, 138, 139
  evaluation of subjective complaints,
    101
  factual basis, 101
  functional disorders,
    emotional factors in, 107
    financial motivation in, 107, 108
    persistence of symptoms
      without change, 105
    recognition, 104-5
    response to treatment, 105

symptoms, 104, 105
Workmen's Compensation
cases, 107, 108
physical therapy, aid in, 126
standard nomenclature, use of, 100
subjective symptoms,
basis for, 104
inconsistencies, 103
manifestations to
defendant examiner, 103
without objective findings, 103
without treatment, 103
Disability,
evaluation of residual, 119, 169
negative attitudes and
orientation, 23
ratings,
subjective vs objective basis, 119
Disc, intervertebral, herniation of,
prognosis after surgery,
speculative complications to
aid attorney, 158-159
signs of, 61
Doctor's role in Medico-legal cases,
importance of, 4, 326
Drugs and Medication,
of pain, 106
dosage in nervous patients, 101
duplicate copies of
prescriptions, 121, 136
evaluation of need, 101
indication of intensity
influence on examination, 25
prescription of, 120
refills, 106, 121, 136

Education, medico-legal, 3
Electroencephalogram,
abnormal patterns, 109-110
interpretations, 109-110
repeated tests, 109-110
Evidence,
surprise claims as cause of
mistrial, 250
Examination,
asymptomatic areas of previous
complaint, 28
back, low, 47-64

flexion, measurement of, 50, 115
functional manifestations, 50
hamstring contractures, 55
hip disease, tests for, 56
measurements, 63-64
motions in standing
position, 54
nerve root irritation, 57
pain over bony areas vs.
ligamentous sites, 116
pelvic tilt, 52, 53
posture, 51
sciatica, tests for, 57
test for veracity of complaints, 116
blood pressure, significance
of, 30, 261
brief general survey, 30
cervical spine, 42
cervigon apparatus for measurement of range of motion, 42-45
complete, including brief general
survey, 30, 81, 261
component parts, 11
defendant
claims of injury or aggravation
by, 92, 303
extensive involvement
and encroachment upon
private practice, 99
false representation of
referral party,
intentional, 97
patient error, 97
receptionist error, 97
harrassment by exposure of
examiner's personal or
professional problem, 95, 96
harassment by plaintiff
attorney, 89, 90
hold file
for identification of
referral party, 98
for medical reports to
be used in evaluation
of plaintiff, 98
hostile patients, 91
letters of complaint
following, 90-92

loss of appointment time
   by "no shows", 225
malpractice actions,
   after, 89-96
necessity and incidence of
   testimony, 99
obnoxious patients, 84
presence of attorney at, 28
presence of treating
   physician at, 29
restriction by court order, 85
   (case report) 85-89
review and abstract
   of medical records, 191
scheduling, 97
trial alerts, 99
   cancellation, 100
   payment for lost professional
     time, 100
x-rays, 81
evaluation prior to settlement, 25
   reassurance prior to settlement, 25
final evaluation,
   deferred for 1 week or more after
     last treatment, 186
grip testing,
   scientific evaluation, 38
   tests for malingering, 41
   variations, 38, 40
inquiries, technique of, 60
lower extremities, 46, 47
malingering,
   (see malingering, 113)
measurements, 37
muscle spasm, voluntary
   vs. involuntary, 46, 114
nervous factors,
   cogwheel motions, 50
neurological, 46
observation of dress as clue to
   actual disability, 26
sensation,
   indicator of functional overlay, 46
   loss of, 46
   vibratory sensation, 46
tenderness,
   consistency with attention

   diverted, 115
   undressed sufficiently for, 26
Examinations, medico-legal,
   cursory, 8
   objective measurements in, 8
   use of dictating apparatus, 8
   use of outline forms, 8
Exhibit, medico-legal,
   frontispiece
Exhibits,
   use of charts, skeletons, etc.
   to reinforce medical
     testimony, 250, 251
Expert Witness,
   cannot be compelled to testify as
     expert without compensation, 275

Fees,
   acceptance of reduced fee, 227
   compensation for excessive loss
     of office appointments, 223
   contingency basis, 199, 203, 227, 228
   defendant testimony, 223
   delayed payment, 224
   depositions, 225, 226
   final bill, sent with final
     report, 198
   itemized bills, 198
   medical examinations
     and progress reports, 198
   medico-legal reports, 197
   padded, 198, 217
   periodic billing,
     notations on bill requesting
       status report, 199
   reduced fee, request of
     plaintiff attorney, 228, 229
     retention of reduced portion of
       doctor's fee by attorney, 228
   regular monthly billing, 217
   testimony and conferences, 198,
     217-219
   testimony as ordinary witness, 226
Forms,
   after-cast care, 134, 316
   assignment and
     authorization, 200, 201, 202
   cervical spine, examination of, 33

chest, examination of, 36
ENT and brief neurological,
  examination of, 35
examination outlines,
  use of, 31
instructive memoranda, 127-136, 316
lower extremities, examination of, 35
lumbar spine, examination of, 34
notation of measurements, 32
outlines for examination, 316
consent forms, 315
Fractures,
  discovery in defendant
    examination, 118
  missed by treating doctor, 118
  notification of treating doctor, 118
Functional disorders,
  see Diagnosis, functional
    disorders, 107
  parenteral influences,
    illustrative case report, 142-144

Gout, 108

Harassment,
  defendant examiner, 89-96, 276, 277
History,
  accidents,
    details, 13
    immediate care and activities, 13
    time and place, 13
    type of impact, 13
    vehicles involved, 13
  ambulance, need of, 14, 17
  braces and supports, use of, 22
    cervical collar, 22, 23
    lumbar support, 22
    need of, 22, 23
    regular use of, 22, 23
  chronological, 12
  complaints,
    initial, 18
    later, 18
    relation to x-rays taken, 18
  complete, 12
  cross-examination on lack of
    familiarity with facts, 16
  defendant examination, 16

denial of known facts, 11
difficulties in obtaining, 16
disability,
  partial, 20
  total, 20
  insurance forms for, 20
fractures,
  details of treatment, 19
hospital care, 17
length, 12
loss of time from work, 20
necessity, 12
nervous problems, 14
  disability awards and pension, 19
  onset after accident, 19
  prior episodes, 19
  systemic manifestations, 19
past medical, 14
previous accidents, 11
probing into legal details, 17
property damage,
  influence on injuries, 16
  pictures of, 16
receptionist's portion of,
  review by doctor, 14
removal from scene of
  accident, 14, 17
treatment,
  areas treated, 21
  frequency, 21
  last date of, 21
  response, 21
  type, 21
unconsciousness, 18
veracity and credibility, 11
Workmen's Compensation cases,
  employee relations, 24
  employee work record, 24
  functional complaints, 24
Hold File,
  for identification of referral party, 98
  for medical reports to be used in
    evaluation of plaintiff, 98
Home care, 125, 126
Hospitalization,
  for build-up of litigation, 137
  for diagnosis, 138
  for physical therapy, 137

for traction, 137
necessity for, 136
Hospital records,
  release to encourage early
    disposal of unfounded claim, 19
  release to patient without
    doctor's authorization, 190
Hostile patients, 91

Impartial medical testimony,
  impact on litigation, 268, 269
  trial project in New York
    City, 267, 268
Injury,
  claims after defendant
    examination, 92, 303
  priority of concern for
    property damages, 109
Instruction sheets,
  exercise routines,
    back, 130, 131
    knee, 133
    neck, 129
    shoulder, 132
  liniment rubs, 125, 135
Insurance benefits,
  Aetna Government-Wide plan, 211
  assignment of supplemental benefits
    of Blue Shield plan, 209, 212
    assignment form, 211
    explanatory memorandum, 210
  assignment to pay doctor, 207
  multiple health and accident
    coverage, 208
  typical assignment form, 208

Judge,
  questioning of witness, 265

Legal actions,
  diversified types, 5
  involvement with physicians, 5
Legal Forms, 315, 316
Liniment, 125, 135

Malpractice,
  claims after defendant
    examinations, 90-96, 303

Malingering,
  complaints, persistent, 112
  detection of, 110-113
  differentiation from hysteria
    and exaggeration, 111
  examination, 113-117
  frequent changes of physicians, 113
  grip testing, Jamar, 113
  history in, 111-113
  repeated injuries after
    minor accidents, 112
  sensory disturbances in, 113
  tests for veracity and authenticity
    of complaints, 113-117
Medical expert,
  qualifications of, 230-231
Medical Pay coverage,
  assignment, 212
  explanatory memorandum, 214
  information required, 212
  proof of claim form, 212
  use to pay doctor's bill, 212
Medical seminars and
  conventions, 235, 255-257
Medico-legal case,
  involvement, 7
  withdrawal, 7
Medico-legal code,
  cooperation of lawyers
    and doctors, 319, 324
  Maryland plan, 319-324
  usefulness and need, 319
Muscle spasm, 46
  voluntary vs. involuntary, 46, 114
Myelogram,
  accuracy, 82
  false positives, 83
  indication and importance, 82, 83

Nerve blocks, 125
Nervous factors,
  relation to organic injuries, 101, 325

Obnoxious patients, 84

Pain,
  emotional factors, 107
  evaluation of, 105-109

psychosomatic vs. physical
pain, 105-109
Pamphlets,
home care of neck and
back injuries, 126, 127
Patients,
uncooperative or hostile, 91
Patients, former,
failure to remember prior visits, 9
importance of previous observations
and reaction to treatment, 10
importance of recognition in
defendant examinations, 10
recognition of, 9
Physical therapy,
check-up examinations, 123
indications, 121
modalities, 121
overtreatment,
illustrative case report, 139-141
unfavorable emotional
reactions, 139
prescription of, 122
use as diagnostic aid, 126
Physician,
attendance at defendant
examination, 29
Prescriptions,
duplicate copies in patient's
file, 121, 136
Prognosis,
causal connection between
pre-existing conditions and
traumatic aggravation, 165, 166
exaggeration of complaints, 166
need for additional treatment, 167
post-operative complications,
speculation to aid
attorney, 152-160
residual disability, 169
return to work, 167, 169
surgical procedures, 152-160

Qualifications,
doctor as a medical expert, 230
recital of, 230, 265
recognition by presiding judge, 231
stipulation by opposing counsel, 231

Records, hospital,
release to patient without
doctor's authorization, 190
Records, medical,
review before testifying, 252
Relations, medical and legal
professions, 324
Reluctance, professional witnesses, 4
Reports, medical
alteration of, 192
credibility of, 169
defendant examination,
after prolonged treatment
and surgery, 179-182
after short course of
treatment, 177,179
dictation in presence of plaintiff
attorney, 129
review and abstract of medical
records, 182-184
dictation during examination, 31
final evaluation,
bill, inclusion of, 186
prognosis, 186
typical report after cervical
injury, 187
typical report after cervical and
lumbar injury, 188
typical report after lumbar
injury, 188
format, 171
forwarding of,
to attorneys in Workmen's
Compensation cases, 195
to opposing attorney, 194
to insurance companies, 194
to patients after evaluation for
Civil Service Commission, 196
full disclosure, 117-118
impartial, 169
importance in the disposition of
litigation, 7, 172
need, 4
omission of unnecessary
statements, 193
plaintiff examination,
typical report of, 173-176
pre-fabricated forms and outlines,

use of, 31
progress reports,
    determination of need of
        additional therapy, 184
    supervision of treatment
        program, 184-185
    typical report of cervical spine
        injury, 185
    typical report of lumbar spine
        injury, 185
prompt dictation of, 172
results of surgery,
    speculation of poor
        prognoses, 152-160, 189, 250
sent to attorney only after receipt
    of countersigned assignment
    form, 204
surgery,
    anticipated costs, 189
    medical basis for, 189
    speculation of poor
        results, 152-160, 189, 250
Reports, status of litigation or settlement,
    cooperation of attorney required, 206
    follow-up phone calls, 205
    illustrative form, 205
    information obtained, 204, 205
    periodic inquiry to attorney, 204
    protection of accounts receivable, 204
    regular billing of patients, 204
    transfer of cases to another
        attorney, illustrative case, 206

Settlement,
    direction negotiation by patient
        without payment of doctor, 216
    medico-legal cases, 326
Subpoena,
    contempt of court citation, 247
    failure to comply with, 247
    testimony in response to, 226
        expert testimony not
            required, 241-245, 271-275
        scope of, 241-245, 271, 275
Surgery,
    fracture of elbow,
        Vitallium prosthesis
            case report, 160-168

in accident prone litigant, 150
    multiple operations, 150-151
influence on settlement, 145, 155
poor prognosis,
    illustrative case reports, 153,
        155, 156, 158
report of results of,
    speculative and catastrophic
        prognosis to aid plaintiff
        attorney, 152-160, 189, 250
shoulder,
    ruptured rotator cuff, 160
significance in medico-legal
    cases, 144-145
unnecessary,
    illustrative case reports, 145-152
    malpractice claims, 145, 146
    need for psychiatric
        evaluation, 150-152
    responsibility of defendant, 145
    significance in plaintiff's
        damages, 88, 89, 144-146
Strain, cervical,
    in women, 108
    treatment,
        exercise instruction sheet, 129
Strain, low back,
    manifestations, 62

Testimony,
    advocate behavior, 251
    appearance at appointed time, 235
    basis of charges for, 218
    cancellation of,
        loss of time by medico-legal
            expert, 220
    comment on qualifications of other
        medical witnesses, 9, 258, 259, 307
    conservation of doctor's time, 221-222
    courtroom manner, 237
    deferment to attend medical
        seminars or vacation, 235, 255-257
    delays in courtroom, 236
    dress and general appearance, 237
    exaggeration of qualifications or
        evidence, 238
    exorbitant fees for, 217
    expert witness in response to

subpoena without fee
  agreement, 226, 241-245, 271-275
fear of court appearances, 233
fees for, 217-219
fees for time lost by settlement,
  cancellation or postponement
  of trial, 219, 220
for opposing counsel, 263
  necessity of subpoena, 263
  result of fair evaluation and
    report, 263, 264
full disclosure,
  confusion of jury by irrelevant
    facts, 260, 261
  relevant vs. irrelevant
    facts, 260, 261
in response to subpoena, 226, 234,
    235, 239, 241-245, 271-275
  compensation, 239
  guidance from judge, 239
    illustrative case, 241-244
  type of evidence given, 239, 240
malingering, 249
  (see Malingering)
observation of cervical collar
  incorrectly worn in
  courtroom, 304, 305
ordinary witness in response to
  subpoena, 226, 239, 241-245,
  271-275
questions by judge, 265
  impact upon jury, 266
postponement to attend medical
  seminar, 235, 255, 257
preparation for, 232
preparation of records, 234
pre-payment of fee, 226
pre-trial discussion of fees, 218
relative weight of different
  specialists, 259-260
relative weight of opinion of treating
  physician vs. single defendant
  examination, 260, 307-311
relative weight of specialists vs.
  general practitioners, 258, 259
reluctance of physicians to become
  medical witnesses, 3-5, 233
signals to attorney, 238

time of court appearance, 235, 236
timely alerts, 221, 222
use of medical records, 252
  removal of embarrassing
    correspondence or notes
    before testifying, 252
voluntary agreement to testify, 246
  legal obligation, 246
  liability to suit for damages for
    non-appearance, 246, 247
volunteered information,
  beyond scope of question, 262
yes and no questions, 238, 306
Tests,
  exaggeration, 36
  malingering, 36, 37
Textbooks,
  recognition of expertise, 284
  use in cross-examination, 283, 284
  validity of opinion based on
    textbooks vs. defendant
    examiner, 284
Treatment, 120-137
  Buck's extension or pelvic
    traction, 124
  cooperation of patient, 27
    significance of failure to
      cooperate, 27
  drugs and prescriptions, 120
  exercise programs, 127-133
  home care, 125, 127, 135
  hospitalization, 136, 137
  instructive memoranda and pamphlets
    for home care, 126-135
  physical therapy, 121-123
  surgery, 144, 145, 160-168

Workmen's Compensation cases,
  functional disorders in, 107-108

X-Rays,
  children, interpretation in, 77
  defendant examinations,
    importance in, 81
    obtain at initial visit, 81
  importance of negative studies, 64
  repetition after time interval, to
    detect undisplaced fractures, 64

loss of lordotic curve, 74, 75
obtaining previous x-rays, 254
osteoarthritis, diagnosis of, 79
    progression of, 68
    traumatic aggravation of, 68
osteophytosis, asymptomatic, 68, 79
release of films and reports from

hospitals, 255
reports from other physicians, 73, 75
reports, needed to institute proper
    treatment, 80
review of prior films, 254, 255
use in courtroom, 252-254
value of negative films, 253, 254